Simulated Patient Methodology

THEORY, EVIDENCE AND PRACTICE

Simulated Patient Methodology

THEORY, EVIDENCE AND PRACTICE

EDITED BY

Debra Nestel PhD, FAcadMEd, CHSE-A

Professor of Simulation Education in Healthcare
School of Rural Health, HealthPEER (Health Professions Education and Educational Research)
Faculty of Medicine, Nursing and Health Sciences
Monash University Clayton, Victoria Australia

Margaret Bearman PhD, BComp (Hons), BSci CertPerfArts

Associate Professor
HealthPEER (Health Professions Education and Educational Research)
Faculty of Medicine, Nursing and Health Sciences
Monash University Clayton, Victoria Australia

WILEY Blackwell

Library of Congress Cataloging-in-Publication Data

Simulated patient methodology : theory, evidence, and practice / edited by Debra Nestel, Margaret Bearman.
    p. ; cm.
 Includes bibliographical references and index.
 ISBN 978-1-118-76100-7 (pbk.)
 I. Nestel, Debra, editor. II. Bearman, Margaret, editor.
 [DNLM: 1. Patient Simulation. 2. Education, Medical – methods. W 18]
 RT51
 610.73 – dc23
                                                    2014023324

A catalogue record for this book is available from the British Library.

Cover image: © Achim Sass/Westend61/Corbis

Typeset in 9/11 PalatinoLTStd by Laserwords Private Limited, Chennai, India

1   2015

Contents

Contributors

Margaret Bearman PhD, BComp (Hons), BSci, CertPerfArts
Associate Professor
HealthPEER (Health Professions Education and Educational Research)
Faculty of Medicine, Nursing and Health Sciences
Monash University
Clayton, Victoria, Australia

Mary Anne Biro PhD, MPH, BA, Grad Cert Academic Practice, RM, RN
Senior Lecturer of Midwifery
School of Nursing and Midwifery
Monash University
Clayton, Victoria, Australia

Felicity C Blackstock BPhysio (Hons)
Senior Lecturer
Department of Physiotherapy, School of Allied Health
La Trobe University
Bundoora, Victoria, Australia

Mollie Burley MRH, RN
Senior Lecturer
School of Rural Health – Department of Rural and Indigenous Health
Faculty of Medicine, Nursing and Health Sciences
Monash University
Moe, Victoria, Australia

Simon JR Cooper PhD, MEd, BA, RGN, FHEA
Associate Professor
School of Nursing and Midwifery
Monash University
Berwick, Victoria, Australia

Hay Derkx MD, PhD
SP Trainer
Faculty of Health Medicine and Life Sciences
Maastricht University,
Maastricht, The Netherlands

Tanya L Edlington BA
Practitioner and Consultant – Simulated Patient
Melbourne, Victoria, Australia

Jennifer H Fisher DNP, WHNP
Associate Professor, Department of Family Medicine
Associate Director, Center for Advancing Professional Excellence
University of Colorado School of Medicine
Aurora, CO, USA

Carol Fleishman PhD, MS
Academic Program Manager, Standardized Patient and Teaching Associates Programs
Johns Hopkins Medicine
Baltimore, MD, USA

Elaine E Gill PhD, BA (Hons), RHV, RGN, Cert Couns
Head of Clinical Communication and Senior Lecturer
King's College London Medical School at Guy's, King's and St Thomas' Hospitals
London, UK

Gayle A Gliva-McConvey
Director, Professional Skills Teaching and Assessment
Sentara Center for Simulation and Immersive Learning
Eastern Virginia Medical School
Norfolk, VA, USA

Pamela J Harvey BAppSci (Physio), MEd
Lecturer in Medical Education
North West Rural Medical Education Unit
School of Rural Health
Monash University
Bendigo, Victoria, Australia

Brian Hodges MEd, FRCPC, PhD, MD
Vice President Education, University Health Network
Professor, Department of Psychiatry
Scientist, Wilson Centre for Research in Education
Faculty of Medicine, University of Toronto
Toronto, ON, Canada

Shirin Irani MD, FRCOG
Consultant Gynaecologist and Honorary Senior Clinical Lecturer
Heart of England Foundation Trust and University of Birmingham
Birmingham, UK

Jane H Kass-Wolff PhD, FNP-BC
Associate Professor of Nursing
College of Nursing at the University of Colorado Anshutz Medical Campus
Aurora, CO, USA

Ernestine Kotthoff-Burrell PhD, RN, BC, FAANP
Assistant Professor of Nursing
College of Nursing at the University of Colorado Anshutz Medical Campus
Aurora, CO, USA

Richard Lawton BA, BComm
Coach and Consultant at Ignite Coaching
Melbourne, Victoria, Australia

Nancy L McNaughton MEd, PhD
Associate Director, Standardized Patient Program
Affiliated Scholar, Wilson Centre for Research in Education
Faculty of Medicine, University of Toronto
Toronto, ON, Canada

Tracy Morrison BAppSci (comp med), MOsteo
Lecturer in Osteopathy
Victoria University
Melbourne, Victoria, Australia

Ged M Murtagh PhD
Senior Lecturer in Clinical Communication
Clinical Skills Centre
St Mary's Hospital
Imperial College London
London, UK

Debra Nestel PhD, FAcadMEd, CHSE-A
Professor of Simulation Education in Healthcare
School of Rural Health, HealthPEER (Health Professions Education and Educational Research)
Faculty of Medicine, Nursing and Health Sciences
Monash University
Clayton, Victoria, Australia

Carol C O'Byrne BSP
Associate Registrar and Manager, Qualifying Examination – Part II (OSCE/OSPE)
Pharmacy Examining Board of Canada
Toronto, ON, Canada

Jim Parle MBChB, DRCOG, FRCGP, MD
Professor of Primary Care
Primary Care Clinical Sciences
School of Health and Population Sciences
University of Birmingham
Birmingham, UK

Shane Pritchard BPhysio (Hons)
Physiotherapist
Monash University
Clayton, Australia

Jan-Joost Rethans MD, PhD
Associate Professor
Faculty of Health Medicine and Life Sciences
Maastricht University
Maastricht, The Netherlands

Karen M Reynolds BA
Manager, Interactive Studies Unit
University of Birmingham
Birmingham, UK

George D Ridgway PhD
Master of Applied Linguistics
Lecturer (Teaching and Learning)
The University of Sydney
Sydney, NSW, Australia

Cathy M Smith PhD
Lecturer, Department of Family and Community Medicine
University of Toronto,
Toronto, ON, Canada

Rosamund Snow PhD
Patient Experience Specialist
Simulation and Interactive Learning Centres
King's Health Partners
London, UK

Pamela J Taylor LACST, BA, Grad Dip Ed M Rur Hlth
Lecturer, Interprofessional Education
School of Rural Health
Faculty of Medicine, Nursing and Health Sciences
Monash University
Moe, Victoria, Australia

Jill E Thistlethwaite BSc, MBBS, PhD, MMEd, FRCGP, FRACGP
Professor of Medical Education
Health professional education consultant Affiliated to University of Technology Sydney NSW, Australia
University of Technology Sydney, Australia

Tanya Tierney BSc (Hons), PhD
Assistant Dean, Clinical Communication Training and Student Welfare
Lee Kong Chian School of Medicine
Singapore

Anna K Vnuk MBBS, DRACOG, FRACGP, MClinEd, EdD
Associate Professor in Clinical Skills
School of Medicine
Flinders University,
Adelaide, SA, Australia

Jeanie M Youngwerth MD
Assistant Professor of Medicine, Director of Palliative Care
University of Colorado School of Medicine
Aurora, CO, USA

Foreword

This book marks a major advance in the scholarship of clinical education. Its skilful interweaving of theory, practice and experience across the world frames the study of simulated patients (SPs) as a domain with its own scholarly identity.

SPs offer a unique contribution to clinical education, opening a window onto a world that is often hidden. At heart of any clinical encounter two people – a clinician and a patient – are held together in a relationship of care. At one level, this relationship seems blindingly simple; at another, unfathomably complex. Its core is the interaction of one human being with another. Many such encounters are private and deeply personal, inaccessible to outsiders. SPs offer a means of entering such closed worlds, of learning to navigate their waters with skill and compassion.

During the fifty years since SPs appeared upon the scene, a huge diversity of approaches has been explored, described and published across the world. Making sense of such diversity is a challenge, and this book provides a much-needed framework. Its combination of academic rigour with down-to-earth practicality is both refreshing and inspiring.

Writing this foreword gives me particular pleasure. As a surgeon, a general practitioner and an educator I have long been convinced of the value of simulation. Yet there has often been a tension between 'technicist' approaches to procedural training and broader conceptions of clinical care. For more than a decade, Debra Nestel and I have explored how these worlds might be brought together.

This book frames simulated patient methodology as scholarship that continues to evolve. Its scope, depth and rigour mark it out as a pioneering contribution, and its editors and contributors bring a fascinating breadth of insights. The book highlights the rich potential of collaboration between clinicians, patients and SPs themselves. I have no doubt that it will become a landmark in the field.

Roger Kneebone
Professor of Surgical Education
Imperial College London

1 Introduction to simulated patient methodology

Debra Nestel and Margaret Bearman
Monash University, Clayton, Australia

Introduction

'Simulation is a technique to replace or amplify real experiences with guided experiences, often immersive in nature, that evoke or replicate aspects of the real world in a fully interactive fashion'(1). This definition by Professor David Gaba, a pioneer of contemporary healthcare simulation, aptly describes simulated patient-based scenarios. A well-prepared simulated patient (SP) has the ability to draw learners into a scenario quickly, achieving deep engagement. Their mere presence usually prompts interactivity.

The terms *simulated* and *standardized* patients refer to largely similar simulation modalities, that is, a *well* person trained to portray a patient. The level of *standardization* varies according to the context in which the SP is placed. In learning settings, standardization is less critical and often its absence can be a feature. The tailoring of SP encounters can be used to meet the needs of individual learners, and also to introduce all the variation that characterizes human beings. In contrast, in summative or high-stakes (graded) assessments, SPs function as the examination question. Therefore, to permit a fair test, the SP must perform *consistently* within the character of the person they are portraying. Embodied in their role is factual information relevant to the clinical encounter. Whereas in Canada and North America the term *standardized patient* is commonplace, in the United Kingdom (UK) and Australia the commonly used term is *simulated patient*. In the latter tradition, simulated patients who perform in high-stakes assessments have their *behaviour* rather than their *being* described as standardized. These are nuanced differences and reflect historical practices. North America has witnessed a strong testing orientation of SP methodology whereas in the UK and Australia the origins are rooted in supporting learning(2). Hereafter, the abbreviation SP is used to refer to either! Several other terms are used to describe the work of SPs and these include expanding roles too (Box 1.1). Our focus is on the role of SPs, although some chapters consider elements of expanded roles and others consider the role of the SP practitioner.

BOX 1.1 Alternative terms used to describe simulated or standardized patients and expanded roles for SPs

- **Role-player** – Sometimes used interchangeably with the term SP and often includes medical, nursing or health professional students as patients.
- **Clinical teaching associate** – Describes SPs who teach specific physical examination (e.g. breast, rectal, vaginal). The focus is on supporting learners in developing psychomotor, communication and other professional skills. This is a highly specialized role.
- **Trained patient** – Sometimes used interchangeably with the term SP and may or may not include a person who is using their experience of a particular illness to play their role.
- **Patient instructor** – May be used interchangeably with the term SP and may include a person who is using their experience of a particular illness to play their role.
- **Incognito or unannounced patient** – An SP who enters real clinical settings (e.g. pharmacy, general practice) with permission but without being identified as an SP – enabling judgements of clinician performance in action.
- **Volunteer patient** – A patient who is sufficiently well to attend teaching sessions. They may simply be themselves in role-play activities (e.g. an

Simulated Patient Methodology: Theory, Evidence and Practice, First Edition. Edited by Debra Nestel and Margaret Bearman.
© 2015 John Wiley & Sons, Ltd. Published 2015 by John Wiley & Sons, Ltd.

Objective Structured Clinical Examination) or they may play the role of another patient.

- **Hybrid patient** – The combination of an SP and a simulator permitting the practice of procedural and operative skills. The concept was first reported by Kneebone *et al.*(15), who described the blending of simulation modalities as 'patient-focused simulation', and is now widely used internationally.
- **Actor patient** – Used interchangeably with the term SP, although it may refer to professional acting skills of the SP.
- **Confederate** – An individual other than the patient who is scripted in a simulation to provide realism, additional challenges or additional information for the learner (e.g. paramedic, receptionist, family member, laboratory technician)(16). The voice of manikins can also be considered as a confederate role.

Adapted from the Victorian Simulated Patient Network, Module 1: An Introduction to Simulated Patient Methodology.

Although healthcare continues to draw on training and assessment practices in high-reliability industries, simulation is likely to become embedded in all stages of education for the healthcare workforce. In the UK, the Chief Medical Officer reported that simulation was one of the top five priorities of the National Health Service in the coming decade(3). With this sort of strategic and high-level vision, simulation is clearly here to stay.

The contemporary history of SP methodology has many drivers. These are well documented and originate from humanistic, educational and external issues(4,5). The imperative of not causing harm to patients is a critical driver(6). However, we must also be aware of the risks to learners and SPs learning and working in this methodology. A theme throughout this book is the role of SPs as proxies for real patients. As such, they represent patient rather than clinician perspectives(7,8). Several chapters identify ways in which this patient proxy role can be strengthened. Some contemporary SP practices constrain the voice of real patients, which limits their potential in offering patient perspectives. We promote approaches that offer authentic patient voices and thereby

contribute to the development of patient-centred and safe care. Recent history is also witnessing better alignment of simulation-based education in health professional curricula, which means that SP practitioners are more likely to be working with other simulation practitioners. This creates exciting opportunities for practitioners of all simulation modalities to learn from each other.

Although the educational settings in which SPs work can vary widely, there are commonalities in simulation practice. Throughout the book, we refer to six phases commonly found in simulation-based educational activities. All are essential to creating effective educational experiences (Figure 1.1). This simulation framework has been adopted in a national training programme for simulation practitioners in Australia(9). The phases enable practitioners to share a common platform for designing and communicating simulation-based education. For the *Preparation* phase, we are referring to all the activities that take place before the session starts – recruiting and training SPs, database management, setting learning objectives, designing scenarios and so on. The *Briefing* phase refers to explaining the simulation process to all participants, including

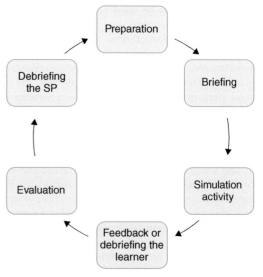

Figure 1.1 Phases in SP-based simulation. *Source: The NHET-Sim Program*, Nestel, D. Module S6: Patient-focused simulation, www.nhet-sim.edu.au (accessed 24 April, 2014). Reproduced with permission of Health Workforce Australia.

the scenario context, learning objectives and the approach to debriefing. Other activities during the briefing may include learners setting their own objectives, sharing prior experience and orientation to the learning environment. There are briefing activities for SPs too, such as checking that they know their role. The *Simulation Activity* is the next phase, and may take different forms, but is where the learner interacts with the SP. The *Debriefing and Feedback* phase follows, which complements the briefing. Learners' feelings are checked, objectives revisited, other perspectives sought and future learning is planned. During the *Reflection* phase, learners (usually individually) are encouraged to make sense of the simulation in the light of their own experience. Similarly, faculty and SPs are also encouraged to reflect on all facets of their contributions. The *Evaluation* phase refers to the success and limitations of the session in meeting its goals, not assessment of the individual. This phase benefits from learner, faculty and SP participation. For SP methodology, there is an 'additional' phase Debriefing the SP before they leave the session. SPs may need assistance in stepping out of their role (sometimes called de-roling) and should leave the session with a sense of their performance and goals for the next encounter. If SPs are undertaking emotionally expressive roles, it can be especially important to de-role and debrief.

Cantillon *et al.* reported on SP programme development in medical education in four European countries(10). Their study sought to establish baseline information for planning regional collaborations. The survey-based study identified minimal sharing of expertise, ideas and scenarios within countries and even less across national borders. There were no consistent approaches to quality assurance in terms of training for role portrayal and feedback to learners. Respondents expressed interest in participating in a network. The cost of SP programmes was seen as a driver to sharing resources insomuch as avoiding duplication of investment in their development and learning 'best practices'. Although the authors acknowledged the challenge in sharing resources across national borders with respect to cultural differences in patients, health professionals and healthcare services, one goal of this book is to share theory, evidence and practice within and beyond the healthcare simulation community.

Unlike other simulation practitioners who work with task trainers, manikins and virtual environments, our simulation *modality* is comprised of real people. As such, we have particular considerations in our practice. One of these is to ensure that SPs are respected and cared for with at least as much respect as the most sophisticated manikin. We have tried to avoid the objectification of SPs(11) by referring to them as co-teachers rather than as objects to be *used*(11).

Although research on SP methodology is rapidly expanding, there are important fundamental areas of practice that have only limited *empirical* evidence, such as methods for effective training of SPs for role portrayal and in offering feedback. However, there is valuable *evidence* that is *experience* and *theory* based. An important example of the latter is incorporation of dramatic and performing arts theory into training methods for SP role portrayal(12–14).

For consistency, we have used the term *learner* to refer to any participant in an educational event. These may be undergraduate students or qualified clinicians. In case studies where specific learner groups are identified, authors have adopted more specific language. The term *faculty* is used to describe anyone involved in working with SPs and could include clinician teachers, facilitators, programme administrators, SP practitioners, educators or trainers. *SP educators* or *trainers*, *per se*, largely do not exist outside the Canada and the United States. The equivalent role is more likely to be incorporated into that of a clinical or communication skills academic role.

Authors in this book share with you their particular journeys and experiences. The book has four parts. The first part, *Foundational Frameworks*, includes the scope of contemporary SP practice through a themed analysis of published literature. An overview of simulation practice is described and then focus shifts to the professional community of the SP practitioner rather than SPs themselves. The second part, *Theoretical Perspectives*, includes an overview of selected theories that underpin SP-based education, before acknowledging the contribution of dramatic arts traditions, the use of a sociological analytic approach – conversational analysis – and finally the role of SPs in the discourses of health professions education. *Educational Practice* is currently the mainstay of SP methodology and as such constitutes the third part. The chapters cover elements of practice across planning, briefing, the simulation activity, debriefing and/or feedback and evaluation. The final part, *Case Studies: Innovations Across the Health Professions*, illustrate creative practice with SPs at their centre. The studies sample across professions, are designed for different levels of learners – undergraduate and qualified clinicians – and in different social and healthcare contexts.

The final chapter reflects on the contents and considers future opportunities and challenges in the theory, evidence and practice of SP methodology.

References

1 Gaba D (2007) The future vision of simulation in healthcare. *Simulation in Healthcare*, **2**: 126–35.

2 Nestel D and Barry K (2006) Association of Standardized Patient Educators. *Medical Teacher*, **28**(8): 746–7.

3 Donaldson L (2009) *150 Years of the Chief Medical Officer's Annual Report 2008*. Department of Health, London.

4 Nestel D, Tabak D, Tierney T, Layat-Burn C, Robb A, Clark S, *et al.* (2011) Key challenges in simulated patient programs: an international comparative case study. *BMC Medical Education*, **11**(1): 69.

5 Bearman M, Nestel D and Andreatta P (2013) Simulation-based medical education. In: Walsh K (ed.) *The Oxford Book of Medical Education*, pp. 186–97. Oxford University Press, Oxford.

6 Ziv A, Wolpe P, Small S and Glick S (2003) Simulation-based medical education: an ethical imperative. *Academic Medicine*, **78**(8): 783–8.

7 Nestel D (in press) Expert Corner: standardized (simulated) patients in health professions education: a proxy for real patients? In: Palaganas J, Maxworthy J, Epps C and Mancini M (eds) *Defining Excellence in Simulation Programs*. Wolters Kluwer: Lippincott Williams & Wilkins.

8 Nestel D and Kneebone R (2010) Authentic patient perspectives in simulations for procedural and surgical skills. *Academic Medicine*, **85**(5): 889–93.

9 The NHET-Sim Monash Team (2012) *The National Health Education and Training-Simulation (NHET-Sim) Program*, www.nhet-sim.edu.au (accessed 29 October 2012).

10 Cantillon P, Stewart B, Haeck K, Bills J, Ker J and Rethans JJ (2010) Simulated patient programmes in Europe: collegiality or separate development? *Medical Teacher*, **32**(3): e106–10.

11 Nestel D, Layat-Burn C, Pritchard S, Glastonbury R and Tabak D (2011) The use of simulated patients in medical education: Guide Supplement 42.1 – Viewpoint. *Medical Teacher*, **33**(12): 1027–9.

12 Sanko J, Shekhter I, Kyle R, Di Benedetto S and Birnbach D (2013) Establishing a convention for acting in healthcare simulation: merging art and science. *Simulation in Healthcare*, **8**(4): 215–20.

13 Wallace P (2006) *Coaching Standardized Patients for Use in Assessment of Clinical Competence*. Springer, New York.

14 Pascucci R, Weinstock P, O'Connor B, Fancy K and Meyer E (2014) Integrating actors into a simulation program: a primer. *Simulation in Healthcare*, **9**(2): 120–6.

15 Kneebone R, Kidd J, Nestel D, Asvall S, Paraskeva P and Darzi A (2002) An innovative model for teaching and learning clinical procedures. *Medical Education*, **36**(7): 628–34.

16 Nestel D, Mobley B, Hunt EA and Eppich W (submitted) Confederates in healthcare simulations: not as simple as it seems. *Clinical Simulation in Nursing*.

Part 1
Foundational Frameworks

2 Scope of contemporary simulated patient methodology

Debra Nestel[1], Tracy Morrison[2] and Shane Pritchard[1]
[1]Monash University, Clayton, Australia
[2]Victoria University, Melbourne, Australia

 KEY MESSAGES

- With training, simulated patients (SPs) are well suited to address diverse learning needs of healthcare professionals, especially those needs related to communication, professionalism and patient safety.
- The scope of SP practices reflects broader trends in healthcare service and education such as teamwork and interprofessional education.

- There is evidence supporting the involvement of SPs in most healthcare professions, at all stages of professional.
- The use of props such as task trainers and body suits together with moulage are extending SP practices for procedural, operative and examination skills.

OVERVIEW

This chapter aims to document contemporary sp practice in role portrayal and the contexts in which SPs work. Drivers for the uptake of simulation influence the ways in which SPs currently work. The main areas for SP practice focus on communication, professionalism and patient safety. The last decade has witnessed the inclusion of SPs in teaching and learning procedural, operative and physical examination skills. Masks, suits and moulage can extend SPs' ability to play different roles. Acknowledging the widening scope of practice, other human-based simulations such as simulated relatives, trainees and healthcare professionals are briefly considered. After a general description of practices, profession-specific applications are outlined, followed by some concluding notes.

Introduction

This chapter explores the scope of contemporary SP practice, acknowledging the impact of social, political and economic factors. Key drivers for SP methodology include the raised profile of patient perspectives – as consumers of healthcare and the acknowledgement that patients experience healthcare differently to those who deliver it(1). Pressures on access to clinical placements have facilitated the expansion of SP-based education.

Quality and safety are dominant themes on any health service agenda(2). SPs can support the development of patient safe practices across all phases of the professional education trajectory. Where patients have been seen as passive recipients of care and contributors to education, SPs can facilitate active and significant roles(1). SPs can also help to address issues of professionalism that are otherwise difficult to access, such as learning to identify and manage ethical dilemmas. The current interest in interprofessional education has

Simulated Patient Methodology: Theory, Evidence and Practice, First Edition. Edited by Debra Nestel and Margaret Bearman.
© 2015 John Wiley & Sons, Ltd. Published 2015 by John Wiley & Sons, Ltd.

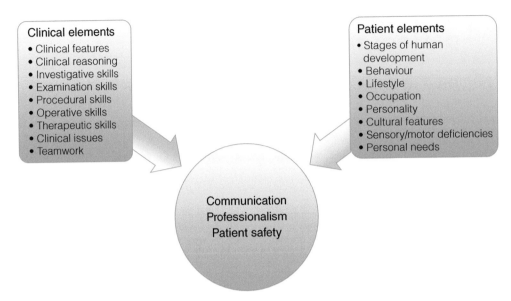

Figure 2.1 Contexts in which SPs work.

led to diverse SP-based simulations to explore interprofessional collaborative practice. National assessments have resulted in the widespread uptake of SP-based testing in which standardized performance by SPs ensures high-quality assessments in clinical skills (see Chapter 12). However, here we focus on the scope of SP practices in role portrayal.

Key elements of learning currently associated with SP-based scenarios include communication, professionalism and patient safety (Figure 2.1). These core components of clinical practice are manifested through scenarios that focus on the information exchange between patients and clinicians including *history taking*, developing management plans and sharing *bad news*. Scenarios may focus on clinical characteristics of illnesses or diseases – acute or chronic – and involve any body system. Aged care and mental health are emerging areas of interest in SP methodology. Trained SPs look, sound and behave as patients with the condition being studied. Clinical reasoning, physical examination, investigative, procedural, operative and therapeutic skills all represent facets of SP-based work achieved through the SP alone or in hybrid simulations. That is, SPs linked seamlessly with task trainers (see below). Clinical issues such as ethical dilemmas, conflict resolution and error disclosure can be explored. Teamwork is another emerging area

for SP-based practice, reflecting a wider interest in team-based approaches to healthcare delivery. These scenarios may be profession specific (e.g. bedside administration of drugs) or interprofessional (e.g. multidisciplinary team meeting, bedside handover). SPs are employed to represent patients with multiple characteristics – across the life span and with different personalities, cultures, life and work experiences, sensory abilities and personal needs.

Integrated approaches to developing clinical skills

Broader changes in clinical skills education have influenced the development of SP practices. Limitations associated with the deconstruction of psychomotor skills into component steps and out of the context in which the clinical skill needs to be practiced (patient and setting) have led to the development of more holistic ways of supporting clinical skills. Here we explore this expanded role portrayal for procedural, operative and physical examination skills.

Hybrid simulations for procedural and operative skills

SPs work in hybrid patient simulations, that is, simulations in which SPs are aligned with

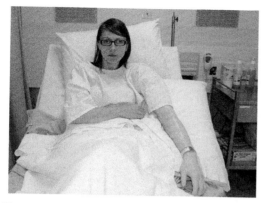

Figure 2.2 Simulator arm aligned with a simulated patient for intravenous cannulation.

simulators designed for learning procedural (e.g. urinary catheterization, cannulation)(3–7), investigative (e.g. endoscopic)(8,9) or operative skills (e.g. carotid endarterectomy)(10). Although the last decade has seen the development of simulators specifically designed for alignment with SPs, many hybrid simulations can be achieved with task trainers (also known as benchtop models) (Figure 2.2).

Training SPs for hybrid simulations requires SPs to gain insight into specific aspects of the clinical task so that they can respond authentically. The concept was developed at Imperial College London(3) in response to the recognition that communication and procedural skills were being taught separately, but in real clinical practice, clinicians had to perform the skills in an integrated manner. Students rarely had the opportunity to rehearse the skills prior to working in real clinical settings. Hybrid patient simulations facilitate this integration and are suited to any clinical skill in which the patient is conscious. If the patient is not conscious, then SPs are probably inappropriate. Even fairly complex procedures are well suited for hybrid patient simulations. If the clinical skill being tested is above the neck, then it is challenging to integrate task trainers with SPs.

Adding realism in hybrid patient simulations

An advance on task trainers being adapted for alignment with SPs is the complete transformation of SP appearance with purposively designed costumes and props. For example, oedema stockings can be worn by SPs to facilitate relevant physical assessment skills(11). Obstetric techniques

are taught in scenarios in which the SP wears a birthing suit. This suit combines a birthing simulator and costume to create a seamless appearance between task trainer and SP (see Chapter 15). The suit has capabilities to exhibit physiological responses (e.g. bleeding) required to address learning goals. In another example, clinicians learn appropriate lifting techniques with SPs who don an obesity suit(11). There are also examples of head and hand masks that can be worn by SPs to create a completely different age and appearance to their own(12). Although not necessarily reflecting a specific pathology, the props enable SPs at least to appear exactly the same as each other. Adhesive wounds are quick and easy solutions to creating signs of trauma(13) (Figures 2.3 and 2.4). In terms

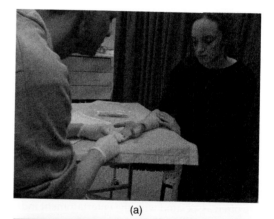

(a)

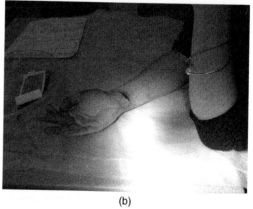

(b)

Figure 2.3 Adhesive wound with moulage for a simulated patient who is self-harming: (a) wide angle and (b) close up. *Source*: Health Cuts Ltd, www.healthcuts.com. Reproduced with permission of Health Cuts Ltd.

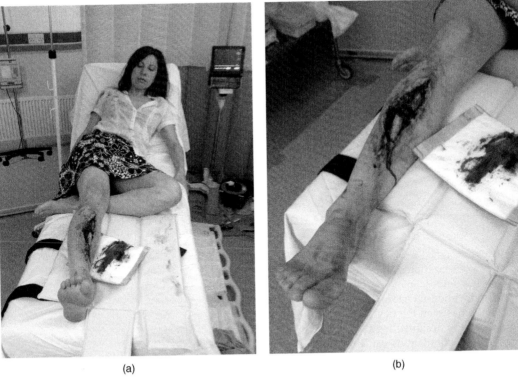

(a)   (b)

Figure 2.4 Simulated patient with adhesive open fracture and moulage: (a) wide angle and (b) close up. *Source*: Health Cuts Ltd, www.healthcuts.com. Reproduced with permission of Health Cuts Ltd.

of appearance, these types of simulators create visual uniformity. Manufacturers of these props are often associated with the entertainment industry. Additionally, SPs participate in simulations that have the trainee using a simulator programmed for a particular response, for example, a stethoscope that provides preprogrammed heart sounds (not the SP's)(14). This permits certainty in terms of the provision of the same clinical cues to learners.

Moulage and SPs

The uptake of moulage in SP-based scenarios is increasing and is facilitated by thoughtful documentation of methods(15). Moulage can provide strong visual cues for cyanosis, pallor, sweating, bruises and pressure areas. Visual and olfactory cues offered through manufactured vomit, blood, urine and faeces together with vapours (e.g. alcohol) add to realism. Although major *disaster* or *first responder* scenarios have used these techniques for

many years, they are becoming mainstream in all SP practices (Figures 2.3 and 2.4).

Physical assessment and examination

Commonly, SPs undergo physical examination as a means of 'testing learners' fundamental clinical skills, especially in medicine students. In these examinations, the actual SP's presentation is that examined by the student. Additionally, since SPs were first reported(16–18), they have been trained to portray physical signs of illness and responses to clinical examinations and tests administered by students. This includes simulating signs from all body systems (e.g. cardiovascular, respiratory, neurological, gastrointestinal, musculoskeletal). Dr Howard Barrows, a pioneer in SP methodology, documented more than 50 signs that SPs can simulate(19). Although this practice continues to develop, others have exercised caution in order to ensure accuracy of presentation. This remains a promising area for developing SP methodology.

Simulated patients in intimate examinations

A specialized form of SP work is that of individuals trained to support learners in developing the skills essential for a range of intimate examinations (e.g. breast, vaginal, rectal, prostate). This is a highly specialized area of SP work. Several terms are used to describe individuals playing this role. Usually these SPs work in pairs and have a significant role as educator of psychomotor, examination and communication skills and professionalism. A case study is presented in Chapter 21.

Simulated patients in expanded settings

SP practices are no longer confined to the simulated consultation room but occur in every clinical setting (e.g. radiography suite, ward, operating theatre, trauma site). Wherever clinicians work, it is feasible that SPs may be found. Innovations in simulated clinical settings, such as photorealistic backdrops to provide visual cues of settings, mean that SPs need to develop awareness of place(20).

Incognito simulated patients

SPs work in real clinical settings. *In situ* simulations in which SPs work *incognito* or *unannounced* have been documented(21). In these simulations, SPs are working in a similar way to the retail concept of *mystery shoppers*, enabling workplace assessments of trainees or clinicians to be performed. Although most examples are in primary care(22–24), there are also examples for interns in the emergency department, for physicians in the detection of sexual risk(25,26) and preregistration pharmacists in pharmacies. A case study is presented in Chapter 16.

Sequential simulations

SPs also work in sequential simulations – a series of related scenarios that often progress through different clinical settings. Sequential simulations often follow a patient pathway in the healthcare service. For example, trainee surgeons may undertake a preoperative assessment and obtain informed consent from a patient. In the second scenario, the trainee may perform a laparoscopic procedure (no SP) in a simulated operating theatre, and the third scenario may involve discharge planning with the SP. The scenarios are usually time compressed, that is, interactions that might usually occur over a few days are presented in one session. A feature of sequential simulations is that students are reconnected with the patient's journey through the healthcare service. This is often lost in current educational programmes with siloed task-focused training. However, there are exceptions to the dominant single episodic model such as a 10-week pharmacy programme in which 'learners interacted with a 'simulated family'(27). Learners had the opportunity to establish and maintain relationships with family members throughout the programme. In another example, learners managed patients with chronic illnesses and this facilitated deeper levels of feedback to learners as the relationships between learners and SPs developed(28,29).

Other simulated roles

The expansion of SP roles challenges the very name *simulated patient*. SPs are taking on additional roles as relatives, trainees, healthcare students and qualified healthcare professionals (30–32). Simulating health professionals has been a common practice in manikin-based simulations where faculty may take on the role of a healthcare professional (e.g. confederate) in a high-technology simulation.

Simulated and real patients

SPs have been described as proxies for real patients and it is important to think about ways in which SPs can get *closer* to real patients. Nestel and colleagues described a process in which SPs worked with real patients in the development of roles, performance and feedback(33–35). In one study, the authors developed the process in order to fill a gap in obtaining complex medical histories for final-year students(34). Many of the scenarios offered to medical students had a single focus aligned with the student's clinical rotation. However, real patients often present with multiple pathologies. In collaboration with clinical faculty, patients with complex histories were invited to participate. The project brought real patients and SPs into close contact. Real patients shared personal and clinical information directly with SPs, which was a new experience for the SPs. The process proved salutary for the SPs, who were reminded in the most compelling way of those for whom they were proxies(36).

Simulated patients in research

The literature documents the role of SPs in research projects with broad-ranging goals, that is, research that is not about the SPs *per se* but about elements of clinical practice such as clinical reasoning(17) and the use of new technologies such as mobile remote presence(37) and telepresence(38).

Profession-specific illustrations

Here we provide specific illustrations of SP practices in medicine, nursing, pharmacy and physiotherapy.

Medicine
Several descriptions and reviews of SP contributions to trainees across the medical professional training pathway have been reported(17,19,23, 39–44). At the undergraduate level, SPs most commonly contribute to supporting medical students in developing patient-centred interviewing skills. However, there is evidence that they contribute to all the areas identified in Figure 2.1. SPs have a critical role in summative assessments in Objective Structured Clinical Examinations.

Nursing
The published literature on the contributions of SPs to nursing education is diverse. SPs have worked with undergraduate, international and advanced practice nursing students and practitioners, in both teaching sessions(45–50) and assessments(51–53). SP scenarios have been reported that address communication skills(46,48, 49), physical examination skills(54,55), safe manual handling(53) and personal care assistance (e.g. providing advice on oral care), hybrid simulation for urinary catheterization and enema administration(53).

Pharmacy
Although SPs are contributing to pharmacy education in the development of trainees' communication skills, patient assessment skills and ability to educate clients, there are also several examples of incognito SPs in community pharmacy consultations(56–59). These include assessments of various pharmacist competencies such as discerning the nature and severity of a problem in order to determine the best treatment or if the presentation necessitates a further opinion and should be referred. Specific studies describe education about asthma(60), counselling skills(61), advice on over-the-counter medications(56) and providing the emergency contraceptive pill(58). SPs were also invited to provide feedback.

Physiotherapy
SPs are contributing to teaching sessions and assessments across musculoskeletal, cardiovascular, respiratory and neurological systems in physiotherapy education. SP scenarios have been developed to facilitate skills development in communication(62), professionalism(63–65), clinical reasoning(63,66) and physical examination(67,68). Randomized controlled trials have demonstrated that substituting 25% of a 4-week clinical placement with SP-based practice resulted in comparable learning outcomes for physiotherapy students compared with those who undertook 'conventional' 4-week clinical placements(67,69). The portrayal of abnormal movement patterns in gait and when transferring patients from different body positions (e.g. lying to sitting to standing and bed to chair) have been achieved by SPs. Demonstrations of the movement disorder, an opportunity to practice it and constructive feedback on their performance are strategies successfully used by SP educators in preparing SPs.

Conclusion

This chapter has documented the scope of contemporary SP methodology. Historical and broader influences on healthcare services and educational practices directly impact current SP practice. Lack of creativity rather than resources may limit the scope of SP practices. Many practices described here are not expensive but are thoughtful responses to limitations in current clinical skills curricula and problems in healthcare. The implications of this widened scope of practice means that SPs and faculty need to consider ways to ensure that SPs are well prepared and cared for as they take on new ways of working. Involving SPs as partners in these developments promises an exciting future.

References

1 Nestel D and Bentley L (2011) The role of patients in surgical education. In: Fry H and Kneebone R (eds) *Surgical Education: Theorising an Emerging Domain*, pp. 151–168. Springer, Dordrecht.

2 Donaldson L (2009) *150 Years of the Chief Medical Officer's Annual Report 2008*. Department of Health, London.

3 Kneebone R, Kidd J, Nestel D, Asvall S, Paraskeva P and Darzi A (2002) An innovative model for teaching and learning clinical procedures. *Medical Education*, **36**(7): 628–34.

4 Kneebone R, Nestel D, Bello F and Darzi A (2008) An Integrated Procedural Performance Instrument (IPPI) for learning and assessing procedural skills. *Clinical Teacher*, **5**: 45–48.

5 LeBlanc VR, Tabak D, Kneebone R, Nestel D, MacRae H and Moulton CA (2009) Psychometric properties of an integrated assessment of technical and communication skills. *American Journal of Surgery*, **197**(1): 96–101.

6 Moulton CA, Tabak D, Kneebone R, Nestel D, MacRae H and LeBlanc VR (2009) Teaching communication skills using the Integrated Procedural Performance Instrument (IPPI): a randomized controlled trial. *American Journal of Surgery*, **197**(1): 113–8.

7 Kneebone R, Nestel D, Yadollahi F, Brown R, Nolan C, Durack J, *et al.* (2006) Assessing procedural skills in context: exploring the feasibility of an Integrated Procedural Performance Instrument (IPPI). *Medical Education*, **40**(11): 1105–14.

8 Kneebone R, Nestel D and Taylor P (2003) Can 'performing' a procedure help students explain it to their patients? *Medical Education*, **37**(5): 481–2.

9 Kneebone RL, Nestel D, Moorthy K, Taylor P, Bann S, Munz Y, *et al.* (2003) Learning the skills of flexible sigmoidoscopy – the wider perspective. *Medical Education*, **37**(Suppl 1): 50–8.

10 Black SA, Nestel DF, Horrocks EJ, Harrison RH, Jones N, Wetzel CM, *et al.* (2006) Evaluation of a framework for case development and simulated patient training for complex procedures. *Simulation in Healthcare*, **1**(2): 66–71.

11 Eriter Creations (2013) *SimLeggings*, http://simleggings.com/ (accessed 5 September 2013).

12 CQUniversity (2013) *Mask-Ed*, http://www.cqu.edu.au/masked (accessed 4 September 2013).

13 HealthCuts (2013) *Realistic Training Models for Medical Simulation*, http://www.healthcuts.com/ (accessed 4 September 2013).

14 Lecat P (2013) *Lecat's Ventriloscope*, http://www.simply-sim.com/ (accessed 4 September 2013).

15 Merica B (2012) *Medical Moulage: How to Make Your Simulations Come Alive*. F.A. Davis Company, Philadelphia, PA.

16 Barrows HS (1968) Simulated patients in medical teaching. *Canadian Medical Association Journal*, **98**(14): 674–6.

17 Barrows HS (1993) An overview of the uses of standardized patients for teaching and evaluating clinical skills. *Academic Medicine*, **68**(6): 443–51; discussion, 451–3.

18 Wallace P (2006) *Coaching Standardized Patients for Use in Assessment of Clinical Competence*. Springer, New York.

19 Cleland J, Abe K and Rethans J (2009) The use of simulated patients in medical education: AMEE Guide No. 42. *Medical Teacher*, **31**(6): 477–86.

20 Kneebone R, Arora S, King D, Bello F, Sevdalis N, Kassab E, *et al.* (2010) Distributed simulation – accessible immersive training. *Medical Teacher*, **32**(1): 65–70.

21 Gordon J, Sanson-Fisher R and Saunders NA (1988) Identification of simulated patients by interns in a casualty setting. *Medical Education*, **22**(6): 533–8.

22 Luck J and Peabody J (2002) Using standardised patients to measure physicians' practice: validation study using audio recordings. *BMJ*, **325**(679): 1–5.

23 Rethans JJ, Gorter S, Bokken L and Morrison L (2007) Unannounced standardised patients in real practice: a systematic literature review. *Medical Education*, **41**: 537–49.

24 Rethans JJ, Drop R, Sturmans F and van der Vleuten C (1991) A method for introducing standardized (simulated) patients into general practice consultations. *British Journal of General Practice*, **41**(344): 94–6.

25 Russell NK, Boekeloo BO, Rafi IZ and Rabin DL (1991) Using unannounced simulated patients to evaluate sexual risk assessment and risk reduction skills of practicing physicians. *Academic Medicine*, **66**(9 Suppl): S37–9.

26 Russell NK, Boekeloo BO, Rafi IZ and Rabin DL (1992) Unannounced simulated patients' observations of physician STD/HIV prevention practices. *American Journal of Preventive Medicine*, **8**(4): 235–40.

27 Austin Z and Tabak D (1998) Design of a new professional practice laboratory course using standardized patients. *American Journal of Pharmaceutical Education*, **62**, 271–9.

28 Linssen T, van Dalen J and Rethans JJ (2007) Simulating the longitudinal doctor–patient relationship: experiences of simulated patients in successive consultations. *Medical Education*, **41**(9): 873–8.

29 Linssen T, Bokken L and Rethans JJ (2008) Return visits by simulated patients. *Medical Education*, **42**(5): 536.

30 Kassab ES, King D, Hull LM, Arora S, Sevdalis N, Kneebone RL, *et al.* (2010) Actor training for surgical team simulations. *Medical Teacher*, **32**(3): 256–8.

31 Nestel D, Black SA, Kneebone RL, Wetzel CM, Thomas P, Wolfe JH, *et al.* (2008) Simulated anaesthetists in high fidelity simulations for surgical training: feasibility of a training programme for actors. *Medical Teacher*, **30**: 407–13.

32 Nestel D, Van Herzeele I, Aggarwal R, Odonoghue K, Choong A, Clough R, *et al.* (2009) Evaluating training for a simulated team in complex whole procedure simulations in the endovascular suite. *Medical Teacher*, **31**(1): e13–18.

33 Nestel D, Cecchini M, Calandrini M, Chang L, Dutta R, Tierney T, *et al.* (2008) Real patient involvement in role

development evaluating patient focused resources for clinical procedural skills. *Medical Teacher*, **30**: 795–801.

34 Nestel D and Kneebone R (2010) Authentic patient perspectives in simulations for procedural and surgical skills. *Academic Medicine*, **85**(5): 889–93.

35 Nestel D, Tierney T and Kubacki A (2008) Creating authentic roles for simulated patient roles: working with volunteers. *Medical Education*, **42**(11): 1122.

36 Nestel D (in press) Expert Corner: Standardized (simulated) patients in health professions education: a proxy for real patients? In: Palaganas JC, Maxworthy JC, Epps CA and Mancini ME (eds) *Defining Excellence in Simulation Programs*. Wolters Kluwer: Lippincott Williams & Wilkins.

37 Nestel D, Sains P, Wetzel CM, Nolan C, Tay A, Kneebone RL, *et al.* (2007) Communication skills for mobile remote presence technology in clinical interactions. *Journal of Telemedicine and Telecare*, **13**(2): 100–4.

38 Krogh K, Gray K and Nestel D (in press) Teleconferencing in rural and remote medical education: focus on TelePresence. In: Chater B et al. (eds) *Rural Guidebook on Medical Education*. Rural and Remote Health.

39 Howley L, Gliva-McConvey G and Thornton J (2009) Standardized patient practices: initial report on the survey of US and Canadian medical schools. *Medical Education Online*, **14**(7).

40 May W, Park J and Lee J (2009) A ten-year review of the literature on the use of standardized patients in teaching and learning: 1996–2005. *Medical Teacher*, **31**: 487–92.

41 Bokken L, Linssen T, Scherpbier A, van der Vleuten C and Rethans JJ (2009) Feedback by simulated patients in undergraduate medical education: a systematic review of the literature. *Medical Education*, **43**: 202–10.

42 Bokken L, Rethans JJ, van Heurn L, Duvivier R, Scherpbier A and van der Vleuten C (2009) Students' views on the use of real patients and simulated patients in undergraduate medical education. *Academic Medicine*, **84**(7): 958–63.

43 Lane C and Rollnick S (2007) The use of simulated patients and role-play in communication skills training: a review of the literature to August 2005. *Patient Education and Counseling*, **67**(1–2): 13–20.

44 Wallace J, Rao R and Haslam R (2002) Simulated patients and objective clinical structured examinations: review of their use in medical education. *Advances in Psychiatric Treatment*, **8**: 342–8.

45 Becker KL, Rose LE, Berg JB, Park H and Shatzer JH (2006) The teaching effectiveness of standardized patients. *Journal of Nursing Education*, **45**(4): 103–11.

46 Eid A, Petty M, Hutchins L and Thompson R (2009) 'Breaking bad news': standardized patient intervention improves communication skills for hematology–oncology fellows and advanced practice nurses. *Journal of Cancer Education*, **24**(2): 154–9.

47 Gillett B, Peckler B, Sinert R, Onkst C, Nabors S, Issley S, *et al.* (2008) Simulation in a disaster drill: comparison of high-fidelity simulators versus trained actors. *Academic Emergency Medicine*, **15**(11): 1144–51.

48 Ramsay J, Keith G and Ker JS (2008) Use of simulated patients for a communication skills exercise. *Nursing Standard*, **22**(19): 39–44.

49 Wakefield A, Cooke S and Boggis C (2003) Learning together: use of simulated patients with nursing and medical students for breaking bad news. *International Journal of Palliative Nursing*, **9**(1): 32–8.

50 Webster D, Seldomridge L and Rockelli L (2012) Making it real: using standardized patients to bring case studies to life. *Journal of Psychosocial Nursing and Mental Health Services*, **50**(5): 36–41.

51 Bolstad AL, Xu Y, Shen JJ, Covelli M and Torpey M (2012) Reliability of standardized patients used in a communication study on international nurses in the United States of America. *Nursing and Health Sciences*, **14**(1): 67–73.

52 Bornais JA, Raiger JE, Krahn RE and El-Masri MM (2012) Evaluating undergraduate nursing students' learning using standardized patients. *Journal of Professional Nursing*, **28**(5): 291–6.

53 Yoo MS and Yoo IY (2003) The effectiveness of standardized patients as a teaching method for nursing fundamentals. *Journal of Nursing Education*, **42**(10): 444–8.

54 Luctkar-Flude M, Wilson-Keates B and Larocque M (2012) Evaluating high-fidelity human simulators and standardized patients in an undergraduate nursing health assessment course. *Nurse Education Today.* **32**(4): 448–52.

55 Vessey JA and Huss K (2002) Using standardized patients in advanced practice nursing education. *Journal of Professional Nursing*, **18**(1): 29–35.

56 Watson MC, Cleland JA and Bond CM (2009) Simulated patient visits with immediate feedback to improve the supply of over-the-counter medicines: a feasibility study. *Family Practice*, **26**(6): 532–42.

57 Watson MC, Skelton JR, Bond CM, Croft P, Wiskin CM, Grimshaw JM, *et al.* (2004) Simulated patients in the community pharmacy setting. Using simulated patients to measure practice in the community pharmacy setting. *Pharmacy World and Science.* **26**(1): 32–7.

58 Weiss MC, Booth A, Jones B, Ramjeet S and Wong E (2010) Use of simulated patients to assess the clinical and communication skills of community pharmacists. *Pharmacy World and Science.* **32**(3): 353–61.

59 Xu T, de Almeida Neto AC and Moles RJ (2012) A systematic review of simulated-patient methods used in community pharmacy to assess the provision of non-prescription medicines. *International Journal of Pharmacy Practice*, **20**(5): 307–19.

60 Dolovich L, Sabharwal M, Agro K, Foster G, Lee A, McCarthy L, *et al.* (2007) The effect of pharmacist education on asthma treatment plans for simulated patients. *Pharmacy World and Science*, **29**(3): 228–39.

61 Horvat N, Koder M and Kos M (2012) Using the simulated patient methodology to assess paracetamol-related counselling for headache. *PLoS ONE*, **7**(12): e52510.

62 Jull G, Wright A, McMeeken J, Morris N, Rivett D, Blackstock F, *et al.* (2010) *National Simulated Learning Project Report for Physiotherapy*. Health Workforce Australia.

63 Black B and Marcoux BC (2002) Feasibility of using standardized patients in a physical therapist education program: a pilot study. *Journal of Physical Therapy Education*, **16**(2): 49–56.

64 Cahalin LP, Markowski A, Hickey M and Hayward L (2011) A cardiopulmonary instructor's perspective on a standardized patient experience: implications for cardiopulmonary physical therapy education. *Cardiopulmonary Physical Therapy Journal*, **22**(3): 21–30.

65 Hayward LM, Blackmer B and Markowski A (2006) Standardized patients and communities of practice: a realistic strategy for integrating the core values in a physical therapist education program. *Journal of Physical Therapy Education*, **20**(2): 29–37.

66 Lewis M, Bell J and Asghar A (2008) Use of simulated patients in development of physiotherapy students' interpersonal skills. *International Journal of Therapy and Rehabilitation*, **15**(5): 221–7.

67 Blackstock FC, Watson KM, Morris NR, Jones A, Wright A, McMeeken JM, *et al.* (2013) Simulation can contribute a part of a cardiorespiratory physiotherapy clinical education. *Simulation in Healthcare*, **8**: 32–42.

68 Ladyshewsky R, Baker R, Jones M and Nelson L (2000) Reliability and validity of an extended simulated patient case: a tool for evaluation and research in physiotherapy. *Physiotherapy Theory and Practice*, **16**(1): 15–25.

69 Watson K, Wright A, Morris N, McMeeken J, Rivett D, Blackstock F, *et al.* (2012) Can simulation replace part of clinical time? Two parallel randomised controlled trials. *Medical Education*, **46**(7): 657–67.

3 The content and process of simulated patient-based learning activities

Jill E Thistlethwaite[1] and George D Ridgway[2]
[1]University of Technology Sydney, Australia
[2]University of Sydney, Sydney, Australia

 KEY MESSAGES

- Simulation design draws from a range of learning theories, such as experiential learning theory.
- Learning outcomes must be defined and simulation activities aligned with these.
- The simulated patients' (SPs) expected levels of performance should be clearly outlined.

- Facilitators need details about the learners and the learning space.
- Feedback to learners involves the triad of peers, SPs and facilitators.
- Evaluation is crucial for future development.

OVERVIEW

In this chapter, we look at the content and process of simulation activities and how these need to be informed by learners' previous knowledge and experience. We stress the importance of defining learning outcomes and their alignment with learning activities. There are practical details for planning, such as number of learners, the learning space available and the skill of SPs required. A timeline guide is important that should be flexible to allow for learners' needs, reflection and repetition. Evaluation and assessment are crucial.

Introduction

SP methodology has much in common with other health professional education methodologies. Attention needs to be given to both content and process (Box 3.1). *Content* is about the desired learning outcomes and their alignment with the planned activity. *Process* focuses on the learners; the learning methods plus how they will learn and achieve the defined outcomes. In the design and planning of simulation sessions, including with SPs, there are learning theories in addition to practical factors to consider (Box 3.2).

Content

Learning outcomes

The current trend in health professional education is to define what learners will have achieved by the end of the activity. For simulations in prequalification environments, including those with SPs, the learning outcomes are predominantly set *a priori* and are derived from the broader curriculum. For more senior learners undertaking professional development, the learning outcomes may be set by the learners themselves, either before or at the beginning of a session. Broader learning goals can

---

Simulated Patient Methodology: Theory, Evidence and Practice, First Edition. Edited by Debra Nestel and Margaret Bearman.
© 2015 John Wiley & Sons, Ltd. Published 2015 by John Wiley & Sons, Ltd.

BOX 3.1 Content and Process Elements of Simulation Sessions

CONTENT

- The defined learning outcomes (how these fit with the rest of the learners' educational programme).
- The learning activities.
- The assessment, if any – whether formative and/or summative.

PROCESS

- The learning theory and methodology including the type of feedback.
- Orientation activities and ice-breakers.
- Briefing and debriefing activities.

BOX 3.2 THE PRACTICAL FACTORS IN SP SESSION DESIGN: What Needs to be Known

- Number and type of learners.
- What the learners already know about the topic(s) to be covered.
- Learners' previous experience of working with SPs (if any).
- Whether the learners have learnt/worked together before.
- The number and duration of sessions.
- The number and experience of the educators/facilitators.
- The learning environment – size and layout of the space.
- Facilities available – tables, flip charts, computer, projector, manikins, audiovisual recording.
- The number, experience and role of SPs required and available.
- Type of briefing and/or training the facilitators and the SPs may need.
- The budget.
- How the session/programme will be evaluated.

initially be set, such as to improve communication/consultation skills, teamwork and other generic outcomes. The more specific outcomes are then derived from the learners' stated needs, meaning that facilitators and SPs need to be flexible in what they can deliver.

Knowledge of the learning outcomes is therefore important when planning content, as is knowledge of the *stage* of learners and their prior learning experiences. Questions to ask are:

- How does this simulation fit with the rest of the programme the learners are undertaking?
- Where in the curriculum does this session take place?
- What do the learners already know about the topic/content?

The learning outcomes are aligned with appropriate and relevant simulation activities that may be achieved by all learners. At the end of a session, the outcomes should be revisited to ensure that they have been covered. They may not have been fully achieved at this point, as further learning may be required, and this should be consolidated by practice following the simulation activity.

Assessment

Formative and summative assessment provides evidence that learners have achieved the learning outcomes and informs both learners and educators that learning has taken place. The alignment of outcomes, activities and assessment resonates with constructivist learning theory and promotes the creation of meaning from the learning experience(1). Not all simulation sessions have a formal assessment component, but they will usually involve feedback that is a type of formative assessment. Formative assessment is now frequently referred to as 'assessment *for* learning'(2), and should involve a discussion between learner and SP and not simply be the giving and receiving of information without dialogue. Learners should be able to use the feedback to plan further learning and practice opportunities. Summative assessment ('assessment *of* learning') may take place at the end of a programme, semester or year depending on how the simulation session fits with the overall curriculum.

Process

Experiential learning

While knowledge is acquired in a number of ways, such as reading or from classroom teaching, the best way to develop skills is to consolidate learning through practice. For the health professions, this means learning through graded experience rather than 'practising on' potentially distressed and vulnerable patients in real-life consultations. Simulation promotes learning by doing and learning by experience. The design of effective SP activities therefore usually includes interaction between learners and between learners and SPs. A learner may move round Kolb's experiential learning cycle(3) in a workplace; however, the process is more controlled within a structured simulation session (Figure 3.1 – modified for a simulation activity). An advantage in learning through simulation is that observation and reflection are not solely an individual process but are enhanced by contributions from group members who advance the skill development of the learner at the focus of the simulation(4). Such social learning resonates with the theories of Vygotsky(5), who posited that a person learns less in individual learning environments but more with guidance and encouragement from experienced colleagues and peers.

The designer and the facilitator need to know if learners are familiar with interactive and group learning, whether they have had experience of role play and/or simulation previously and if they

have learnt and/or worked together before. Such information helps guide the need for orientation and 'ice-breakers', which are activities at the start of a session to help learners become acquainted and feel comfortable working together.

Reflection on the simulation during and after the learning activity helps to link the theory of communication to practice. Learners may need time-outs so that they can recollect from theory or previous learning the appropriate response to a challenging interaction. Inexperienced facilitators often pack too much into a session, underestimating the time needed for discussion around the simulation activity itself. The value of the simulation learning environment is that learning prompts, which aid recall and performance, may come from all of facilitators, peers and SPs. Time for reflection and repetition must therefore be included.

In particular, time for debriefing towards the end of each session is vital. Learners and SPs need to come out of role for adverse emotions to be identified and defused. Debriefing may locate problems or issues identified by SPs but perhaps not noticed by the facilitator. Further time is usually required to debrief the SPs after the learners have left. This may involve easing the SP out of a role, particularly if it included emotionally challenging or intimate situations such as dealing with aggression, breaking bad news or inappropriate drug seeking. Additionally, extra time may be needed to discuss the session itself, plan further sessions to extend the learning outcomes and to consider how the session may be improved in the future.

Learning activities

In general, more inexperienced learners require more structured activities than experienced learners. However, facilitators and SPs need to be prepared to respond to unexpected events and emotions. Although it is useful to have a timeline for the simulation, it is better to use it as a guide rather than detail the minutes required for each component. This has the benefit of allowing the learner to control the pace of the session and practice a skill with more or less depth. An example of a generic simulation session, lasting 2.5 hours with an approximate time guide, is given in Box 3.3.

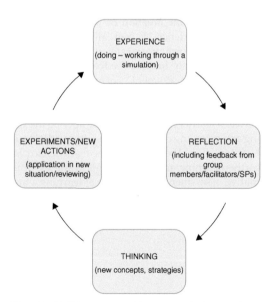

Figure 3.1 Kolb's experiential learning cycle(3) as applied to a simulation activity.

BOX 3.3 Experiential Learning Sessions with SPs – An Example

- Introductions and learner expectations (10 minutes).
- Intended learning outcomes – defining others as necessary depending on learners (10 minutes).
- Setting the scene – overview of the educational activities (5 minutes).
- Orientation to simulation/ice-breaker as appropriate and relevant (15 minutes).
- The experiential learning model (5 minutes).
- Update of any theoretical knowledge required (based on what learners already know) (10 minutes).
- Simulated learning activities with time for debriefing by facilitator and SPs and reflection after each (~20–30 minutes each with a short break between – this is very dependent on the scenarios).
- Discussion and feedback in relation to the whole of the activities (15 minutes).
- Revisiting the learning outcomes (5 minutes).
- Planning the next stage of learning (10 minutes).
- (Assessment).
- Evaluation (5 minutes).

Working with learners who are experienced in simulation reduces the need for too much structure and allows facilitators to change activities to meet specific needs articulated at the start of the session. Health professionals learning together bring a wealth of their own clinical experience to share, and this experience may be utilized to form the basis of learning. A learning activity is more powerful if based on a recounted example from a group learner. When information is sent out to learners about the session they may be asked to give details of any particular scenarios they would like to work with. This allows time for planning and ensuring that an SP of appropriate age or gender is available. However, an experienced facilitator and SP will be able to work through an example volunteered on the day with very little preparation.

Practical considerations affecting design

The learners

All manner of learners may participate in a simulated learning session involving SPs. They may range from junior students to very senior and experienced clinicians. There may be a mix of professions (interprofessional learning) and a diversity of experience and expectations. It is imperative to know the number, designation and experience of the learners in order to develop suitable scenarios. The ideal situation is that all learners will have an opportunity to take part in a simulation. If there are consecutive sessions rather than a one-off activity, there is more flexibility to promote equitable participation. If the group has not worked together before, more time will be needed for introductions and for setting ground rules. If none of the learners have worked with SPs before, more time will be needed for explaining methods.

The simulated patients

The design of activities may be constrained by the number and type of SPs available. Paid rather than volunteer SPs are a budget cost that needs to be considered at an early stage. Part of the simulation may require manikins and other equipment. By knowing the extent of SP involvement, it is easy to factor in their time and, if money is constrained, ensure that when they are on-site they are involved in the activities and not waiting.

Depending on the experience of the SPs, time for their training needs to be included and decisions made on how they will be involved in planning, evaluation and assessment. When recruiting experienced SPs, the level at which they will be working with respect to role portrayal, feedback and facilitation needs to be specified to achieve the right mix of skills. Drawing from Thistlethwaite and Ridgway[6], levels of practice might be as follows:

- Plays a well-developed role with a detailed script (this is common for summative assessments); does not give feedback.
- Plays a well-developed role with fairly detailed script; gives feedback out of role in facilitator-led session.
- Plays a well-developed role; gives feedback out of role in facilitator-led session.

- Able to adapt role depending on interaction and learning outcomes – does not need well-developed script.
- Able to develop role in a session in partnership with learners based on their experiences.
- Can change the feedback mode to suit the desired learning outcome.
- Plays a well-developed role for an examination; marks candidate only in relation to communication skills or similar.
- Plays a well-developed role for an examination; marks candidate on content using pro-forma, no other observer/assessor present.
- Able to facilitate a small group within a session.

The venue/learning space

As simulation learning is interactive and potentially noisy, a large, level-floored room is required. It is difficult to stage simulations in banked lecture theatres, but we have had experience of successfully running simulations in a large hotel conference room with nearly 100 learners, an expert facilitator and one experienced SP. Little equipment is usually required. SPs can provide accessories such as clothing, cans of alcohol or bandaging for an injury. The facilitator provides examination cards that indicate the findings if the scenario involves a physical examination but which is not carried out in the session. For example, if the scenario involves a patient with a cough, the examination card may read: temperature – normal; pulse – 75 regular; BP (blood pressure) – 130/80; chest – clear.

A computer and data projector may be useful. Video equipment with playback potential is helpful to review performance and enhance feedback but is not always necessary. State-of-the-art consultation rooms with video or one-way mirrors limit the number of learners but are useful for certain higher-fidelity scenarios. Multiple rooms are required for assessments, with ease of flow for candidates between them.

Scenarios and roles

In this chapter, we are considering generic design principles rather than specific scenarios. However, there are principles that enhance the quality of the learning experience and educational impact.

SP roles should be as authentic as possible and based on the defined learning outcomes and learners' prior knowledge and experience. However, it

must also be remembered that the interactions are simulated and will always have some artificiality due to location, timing, observation or breaking down encounters into smaller chunks to match particular learning outcomes. SPs can also come in and out of role as required, but this need not limit the authenticity of learning, if it has been explained to the learners in the briefing.

To help achieve authenticity, roles are best based on real-life patient (or other learner) encounters (see Chapter 9). All health professionals have a bank of encounters on which to draw. While the simulation may only involve a snapshot of the whole story, knowing the short- and long-term outcomes is helpful. These stories only give the professional viewpoint. The SP who helps develop the role may be able to offer different insights into the portrayal from the perspective of the patient or other type of role such as family member, student or health professional. Real patient histories may often seem unbelievable, so informing learners that the scenarios are based on real life reduces their 'soap opera' nature. Care needs to be taken that patients cannot be identified from roles, so some aspects of the real story may need to be changed. Alterations to roles may be required if a suitable SP is unavailable, such as approximate age or gender.

Educators frequently have a bank of scenarios with SPs experienced in those roles. It may be necessary to develop new roles or adapt old ones to fit the needs of the sessions, learners and learning outcomes. SPs may need training in new roles, time that needs to be factored into the budget and timeline. A training session may also be needed if the SPs have not worked with this particular type of learner before. Experienced SPs may be able to develop a role from an outline themselves and training may not be needed, although the facilitator and SPs should meet prior to the start of the session to ensure that all are confident about the process.

Timing and pacing the session

As mentioned above, a timeline is useful but needs to be flexible. Timings are certainly important if there are multiple parallel activities and the SPs and/or learners have to move from location to location. Obviously, during formal, usually summative assessments, the timetable will be strictly monitored by a dedicated timekeeper. For other highly structured sessions, the facilitator(s) needs to keep to time. The most important times are the start and finish of the overall session. Starting late can ruin the credibility of the whole process and running over time can cause anxiety. Punctuality also models professionalism.

Evaluation

Thought needs to be given to the type and timing of the evaluation. There may be a standard institutional evaluation form. However, this may not capture what the designers, facilitators and SPs want to know about the session. Evaluation explores whether a learning session or programme has been educationally useful and what its impact has been or may be. Evaluation may take the form of a group discussion at the end of the session or may be more formal with written evaluation questionnaires. Short-term evaluation on the day does not allow learners time to reflect on what they have learnt. Longer-term evaluation is useful to find out what knowledge and skills learners have retained and to ascertain if what they have learnt has been put into practice. If there is intent to publish evaluation data, then relevant ethical approval must be obtained prior to data collection.

Evaluation usually focuses on the outcomes of the educational intervention. A common model of outcomes evaluation is that of Kirkpatrick and Kirkpatrick(7), which provides four types of outcome data. These help designers consider what it is they want to evaluate and what will be useful to help plan further sessions as a quality improvement exercise. Examples of evaluation questions matched to these levels are the following:

I. **Learner reaction and satisfaction:** Did the learners enjoy the sessions? Were the scenarios relevant for their learning and experience? Did they have enough opportunity to participate? Was there enough feedback and was this useful?

II. **Learning outcomes – acquisition of knowledge and skills:** Did the learners achieve the learning outcomes?

III. **Performance improvement and behavioural change:** Will the learners change their behaviour as a result of the activity?

IV. **Patient/health/education outcomes:** These are the most difficult to evaluate and are often omitted.

Outcomes measures are frequently based on self-assessment of change, particularly the types of questions asked at Kirkpatrick levels I and II. More objective measures include pre- and post-intervention assessments of skills, work-based assessment of performance such as the mini-CEX and/or multisource feedback, patient or student satisfaction scores for longer term evaluation of practitioner and educator performance. Realist evaluation takes a different approach: what works, for whom, in what circumstances, in what respects, to what extent and why?(8). This method also explores both unwanted and wanted effects – neither of which may be obvious with standard outcome measures.

Conclusion

Learning outcomes can be derived from the curriculum or a needs analysis. Learning outcomes should be discussed and identified before the simulation begins, to ensure they can be met. More structured and controlled simulations can be created for junior learners or for the purpose of assessment. Much richer and open simulations are available for complex learning needs. During the process of reflection on the simulation, a triad comprised of peer, SP and facilitator can assist the learner to link the theoretical models underlying the learning outcomes to improve performance practice. For a successful learning experience, all learners need to engage positively with the experience and demonstrate acquisition or change of skills and knowledge. Evaluation is important in quality assurance of learning activities.

References

1 Biggs JB and Tang C (2007) *Teaching for Quality Learning at University: What the Student Does*, 3rd edn. McGraw-Hill/Society for Research in Higher Education and Open University Press, Maidenhead.

2 Boud D and Falchikov N (2007) *Rethinking Assessment in Higher Education: Learning for the Longer Term*. Routledge, Abingdon.

3 Kolb DA (1993) The process of experiential learning. In: Thorpe M, Edwards R and Hanson A (eds) *Culture and Processes of Adult Learning*, pp. 138–57. Routledge, Abingdon.

4 Elwyn G, Greenhalgh T and Macfarlane F (2001) *Groups. A Guide to Small Group Work in Healthcare, Management and Research*. Radcliffe Medical Press, Abingdon.

5 Vygotsky LS (1978) *Mind and Society: the Development of Higher Psychological Processes*. Harvard University Press, Cambridge, MA.

6 Thistlethwaite JE and Ridgway G (2006) *Making It Real. A Practical Guide to Experiential Learning*. Radcliffe Medical Press, Abingdon.

7 Kirkpatrick D and Kirkpatrick J (2006) *Evaluating Training Programs: the Four Level Model*. Berrett-Koehler, San Francisco.

8 Pawson R and Tilley N (1997) *Realistic Evaluation*. Sage, London.

4 Communities of practice and simulated patient methodology

Debra Nestel[1], Jan-Joost Rethans[2] and Gayle A Gliva-McConvey[3]

[1]Monash University, Clayton, Australia
[2]Maastricht University, Maastricht, The Netherlands
[3]Eastern Virginia Medical School, Norfolk, USA

 KEY MESSAGES

- Simulated patient (SP) practitioners have responsibility for all facets of SP practices, although position descriptions vary with local requirements.
- SP practitioners currently have no obvious career pathways.
- Professional associations, networks and societies play an important role in the development of SP practitioners.

- The theoretical concept of communities of practice offers a valuable lens through which to view the development of professional identity and expertise.

OVERVIEW

The aim of this chapter is to explore the professional development of SP practitioners, also referred to as educators or trainers. SP practitioners have responsibility for all facets of SP-based teaching and assessment activities. There are currently no obvious career pathways for SP practitioners. We use the theoretical concept of communities of practice to consider how professional associations influence the development of their professional identity and practices.

This chapter draws on the historical context of SP methodology, exploring areas of intersection and distance from the wider healthcare simulation community. Although recent history is witnessing alignment of simulation modalities, SP methodology has often been isolated from other simulation and educational practices. The expansion of SP practices has seen the development of professional associations with SP-based education central to their mission.

Introduction

Who are SP practitioners (educators or trainers), what are the pathways into practice and how do they develop expertise? This chapter seeks to answer these questions. We describe SP practitioners as individuals whose responsibility is to manage all (or part) of SP-based teaching and assessment activities (Box 4.1) and reflected in the simulation phases set out in Figure 1.1. Despite the breadth and complexity of this role, there are currently no obvious formal career pathways for SP practitioners. We use the theoretical concept of communities of practice(1,2) to view the role of professional communities in supporting the development of professional identity and practices of SP practitioners. We document the emergence of SP practitioner communities locally, nationally and internationally.

Simulated Patient Methodology: Theory, Evidence and Practice, First Edition. Edited by Debra Nestel and Margaret Bearman.
© 2015 John Wiley & Sons, Ltd. Published 2015 by John Wiley & Sons, Ltd.

BOX 4.1 SP Practitioner Roles

- **Working with SPs**
  - Recruitment and selection
  - Scenario development
  - Training for role portrayal
  - Training for feedback
  - Moulage

- **Educational administration**
  - Booking SPs
  - Booking facilitators
  - Dissemination of session materials (e.g. SP roles, faculty instructions, rating forms, evaluation forms)
  - Exam preparation and implementation, including security
  - Management of assessment data
  - Designing and collating evaluations

- **Working with clinicians**
  - Scenario development
  - Faculty development activities for working with SPs, including briefing, use of audiovisual review, feedback and debriefing skills
  - High-stakes assessments (e.g. OSCEs)

- **Working with students**
  - Conducting SP-based sessions – formative and summative assessments

- **Programme management and administration**
  - Budgets
  - Payments
  - Communication strategy for programme
  - Databases
  - Facility maintenance
  - Compliance

- **Research**
  - Writing grants
  - Preparing ethics applications
  - Collecting data
  - Writing papers

Describing the work of SP practitioners

There is no singular position description for an SP practitioner. The scope of the SP practitioner role is outlined in Box 4.1. However, the role is usually determined locally and can include programme and educational management and administration (Box 4.2), including quality assurance. SPs practitioners can also work directly with clinicians in scenario development, faculty development and high-stakes assessments. SP practitioners work with SPs in recruitment and selection, in training SPs for role portrayal and feedback and in scenario development. SP practitioners also work with

 BOX 4.2 Examples of Dimensions of Communities of Practice for SP Practitioners

Joint enterprise
- Identifying standards for high-quality SP practices
- Offering of high-quality educational experiences for students and trainees
- Raising patient perspectives in health and social care professional education
- Making judgements of competence of students and trainees

Mutual engagement
- Participating in workshops and other meeting opportunities
- Participating in formal networks (e.g. online discussion boards)
- Collaborating in development of workshops for conferences
- Collaborating in crafting of resources (e.g. SP scenarios)
- Collaborating in research including multisite studies

Shared repertoire
- Terms to describe practice (e.g. scenarios, scripts, roles, brief)
- SP-based scenarios
- Recruitment and selection of SPs
- Training SPs for role portrayal
- Training SPs for offering feedback

students in the implementation of SP-based sessions such as formative and summative assessments. They may also be involved in the development and implementation of SP-associated research projects. This is a diverse range of tasks demanding a broad knowledge base. There are national differences also in the use of the term. In the United States and Canada, the term *SP educator* is well established, whereas in the United Kingdom (UK) and Australia the term is rarely used. Instead, education-focused work outlined above is often undertaken by communication skills academics, while broader clinical skills teams develop and implement examinations such as the OSCE. Not surprisingly, SP practitioners have diverse backgrounds and include, but are not limited to, clinical practice (especially nursing), psychology, performing arts and education. SP practitioners often have a leadership role within the SP programme.

A theoretical concept of communities of practice

Lave and Wenger described a theoretical community of practice as loosely characterized by groups of people working together(1,2). Learning occurs through social practice with participation crucial. Wenger also described three dimensions of communities of practice: joint enterprise, mutual engagement and shared repertoire(2). *Joint enterprise* refers to the agreed goals of the community. *Mutual engagement* refers to the opportunity that members have for participating in community activities – those that further the goals of the community. *Shared repertoire* describes the activities and elements of the community that engender the defining elements of the community. Additionally, Lave and Wenger described the concept of *legitimate peripheral participation*, in which 'newcomers' and 'old-timers' interact. Newcomers undertake meaningful but peripheral tasks in the community of practice that become progressively more complex and central as they gain experience. An important feature of the community of practice is its role in the development of the identity of members and their sense of belonging. Identity is achieved through participation in the community. It includes learning *from* talk and learning *to* talk in the community, thereby highlighting the important role of language(3).

The concept of communities of practice was developed in the context of workplace-based learning, so application to the role of professional associations, societies and networks is an appropriation beyond its original context. However, the dimensions still provide a valuable lens through which to view the development of SP practitioners as a community of specialized practitioners.

Box 4.2 offers examples of the three dimensions of communities of practice for SP practitioners. For *joint enterprise*, this is likely to include creating and upholding standards for high-quality SP practices and raising patient perspectives in health and social care professional education. For *mutual engagement*, this includes the opportunity to participate in workshops, formal and informal networks and collaborating in offering these activities, crafting resources (and thereby contributing to the shared repertoire) and in research activities. Finally, for *shared repertoire*, this includes the specialized language of the community, SP-based scenarios, selection, recruitment and training processes and other practices relevant to the community.

The professional communities appear to operate by offering opportunities for SP practitioners to participate in a range of formal and informal interactions in workshops, discussion boards and other activities. SP practitioners (newcomers and old-timers) undertake meaningful activities in the community of practice. That is, activities that reflect the joint enterprise (e.g. workshops on setting up an SP programme or on giving feedback to SPs). There is a sharing of experiences and resources with the intention of advancing the practice of SP practitioners. Workshops are often facilitated by old-timers in the community and then joined by newcomers as they gain more experience. This seems to be a critical phase in the development of SP practitioner expertise. A recent study by Nestel *et al.* explored the practices of SP practitioners, specifically the ways in which they developed their expertise(4). The dominant process for professional development was participating in workshops at conferences (as newcomers or old-timers).

With respect to the development of identity, professional associations contribute substantially. This is especially important for SP practitioners since there is no obvious career pathway and becoming an SP practitioner may mean shedding a pre-existing identity. The recent certification of healthcare simulation practitioners (a generic role) by the Society for Simulation in Healthcare (SSH) is a step towards acknowledging standards of practice and specialized skills of healthcare simulation practitioners, but it does not necessarily embrace the sense of membership that an SP practitioner may feel to their professional association or network.

Professional communities and simulated patient practitioners

Simulation as an educational method has expanded exponentially in the last decade(5,6). With this expansion, there has been parallel development and/or growth of professional associations, societies and networks. SP practitioners often work in isolation from those performing similar tasks, which is a significant constraint on professional development. There are professional communities that have SP-based education central to their mission, whereas others have a broader goal and membership. SPs themselves are not well represented in these professional communities. There are several reasons for this, an important one being that most SPs are part-time employees or volunteers. Usually SPs are provided with development opportunities locally. Further, there is a financial commitment for participating in many activities, which may prohibits SPs from participating. We acknowledge that Table 4.1 is not an exhaustive list of professional communities but samples across those in which the authors practice.

Simulated patient practitioner communities

The Association of Standardized and Simulated Patient Educators (ASPE) is an international association for professionals in the field of SP methodology that aims to promote best practice for education, assessment and research, dissemination of SP research and scholarship and advancing professional knowledge of SP practitioners through interactivity (Table 4.1). Using the communities of practice dimensions, most SP practitioners are likely to have at least some of these aims with respect to their work (joint enterprise). ASPE seeks to achieve the aims in several ways. The association provides opportunities for participation, including an annual conference,

online seminars, newsletters and a website. Membership of ASPE includes SP programme directors, practitioners and SPs. A current focus of activity is the definition of standards for SP practitioners.

In the UK, there is a network called the Simulated Patient Organizers and Trainers (SPOT), which also has a blended SP practitioner and SP membership. It is noteworthy that membership is free. The website offers minimal information and reports an annual meeting. The Victorian Simulated Patient Network (VSPN) in Australia offers a website with a repository of information on SP methodology. Membership is free and, although extensive resources are provided, it does not currently have capacity for significant online interaction. However, the VSPN offers regional workshops enabling SP practitioners and others to share experiences. In The Netherlands and Belgium, a committee of individuals working with SPs has established a simulated and standardized educators national working committee. This committee serves now under the Dutch Society for Medical Education (~1000 members). Eligibility for this SP committee is associated with representation from all Dutch-speaking medical schools in The Netherlands and Belgium.

Healthcare simulation communities

There are several professional associations, societies and networks for simulation practitioners. One of the largest is the Society for Simulation in Healthcare (SSH), a US-based international association with strong origins in anaesthesia, manikin-based simulations and patient safety. SSH hosts the largest healthcare simulation conference annually and has affiliations with ASPE (and other associations). Although SP methodology has a low profile in keynote presentations at the conference, there are opportunities for SP practitioners to develop their practices by sharing experiences with those who use other simulation modalities. There are also indirect references to SPs through assessments (e.g. OSCEs) and related practices such as confederates in immersive simulations. Preconference workshops cater for SP practitioners. The formal affiliation with ASPE ensures targeted professional development opportunities for SP practitioners. The journal *Simulation in Healthcare* also publishes SP-based peer-reviewed papers.

Table 4.1 Examples of professional associations and networks supporting SP educators.

Association, description and web link	Vision/mission/objectives	Activities
Association of Standardized Patient Educators (ASPE) http://www.aspeducators.org/ An international association for educators interested in the simulated/standardized patient methodology Number of members: 501	• Promote best practices in the application of SP methodology for education, assessment and research • Foster the dissemination of research and scholarship in the field of SP methodology • Advance the professional knowledge and skills of its members • Transform professional performance through the power of human interaction	Website E-blasts Newsletter Peer-reviewed journals: SSH and INACSL Annual conference Research grants
SPOT http://www.spots-online.co.uk A UK-based group of individuals interested in SP methodology Number of members: 14	• Share SP practices • Provide a web-based communication channel for those interested in SP practices	Website for exchanging information Annual meeting
Victorian Simulated Patient Network (VSPN) http://www.vspn.edu.au A state-based network for individuals interested in SP methodology Number of members: 320	• Develop a sustainable network for faculty in SP methodology across Victoria • Provide the highest quality resources for SP methodology • Provide an in-person forum for sharing experiences and demonstrating best practices • Expand SP-based education across the state • Increase the number of simulation educators, in the guise of simulated patients, across the state • Improve education in patient-centred care across the state	Website Online modules Workshops
Dutch/Belgian Working Committee on Simulated and Standardized Patients http://www.nvmo.nl/werkgroepen/simulatie_en_gestandaardiseerde_patienten [in Dutch] This committee is part of the Dutch Association of Medical Education and membership eligibility is associated with representation from medical school Number of members: 25	• Promote human simulation in the widest sense (education/research) • Exchange experience, to promote teaching, to promote research in and with simulated and standardized patients	Three annual meetings
Society for Simulation in Healthcare (SSH) http://www.ssih.org/Interest-Groups/Standardized-Patient-SIG A US-based international society for healthcare simulation practitioners Number of members in Special Interest Group: 101	• Promote, educate and support SPs in all types of simulation supporting the goals of SSH in healthcare education, assessment and research • Publish state-of-the-art SP education methodology in SSH journal • Define standardized/simulated terminology and methodology • Advise and educate members of healthcare systems who are interested in standardized patients/simulated patients • Provide recommendations for high-quality training/simulation • Provide expertise and knowledge to support and develop SP programs, hybrid simulation, design and management of simulation events	Webinar SSH Journal Annual conference

(continued)

Table 4.1 (*Continued*)

Association, description and web link	Vision/mission/objectives	Activities
Society in Europe for Simulation Applied to Medicine (SESAM) http://www.sesam-web.org A European society targeting at all healthcare professionals interested in simulation; no specific SP interest group Number of members: 644	• Develop and apply simulation in education, research and quality management in medicine and healthcare • Facilitate, exchange and improve the simulation technology and knowledge throughout Europe • Establish combined research facilities	Website Newsletter Annual meeting
Australian Society for Simulation in Healthcare (ASSH) http://www.simulationaustralia.org.au/divisions/message-from-the-assh-chair A national society for individuals interested in all facets of healthcare simulation and has an SP special interest group (SIG) Number of members in Special Interest Group: 45	• Develop standards of practice regarding the key applications of simulation, including education, research and patient care • Foster a network of professionals working within the simulation field • Advocate for continued development and availability of simulation-based modalities for key applications including education, research and patient care • Form affiliations with societies and groups having common goals in relation to simulation and safety and quality in healthcare • Promote the professional development of individuals working in the simulation field • Advise on legislation related to the use of simulation in healthcare • Be recognized as the official representative of these groups within Australia	Website Rolling news Annual conference Regional meetings
SimOne http://www.sim-one.ca A provincial-based network in Canada that advocates for and advances simulated learning in health professions education for the benefit of patient care and patient safety Number of members: 950	• Become a strong value-added presence in the simulation field • Move towards achieving self-sufficiency • Advance simulated clinical learning - a critical component of healthcare teaching and learning in Ontario • Expand interprofessional education aligned with interprofessional care • Improve quality of patient care and patient safety • Lay the foundations for further innovation and commercialization of simulation-related intellectual property • Gain a concrete understanding of the results of previous capital investments and maximizing value and return on investment on current and future investments in simulation centres in Ontario	Website Networking events
Association for Simulated Practice in Healthcare (ASPiH) http://www.aspih.org.uk Merger of the National Association of Medical Simulators and the Clinical Skills Network Number of members: 450	• Enable sharing of knowledge, expertise and educational innovation related to simulated practice across healthcare professions • Provide an effective communication network for those involved in simulated practice in the UK and beyond • Provide quality exemplars of best practice and evidence of impact linking simulated practice with improvements in patient safety and quality of care • Develop and share key operational and strategic resources for members drawn from experience within the association from links with relevant educational bodies nationally and internationally	

Table 4.1 (*Continued*)

Association, description and web link	Vision/mission/objectives	Activities
	• Encourage and support scholarly development and recognition of members through wider dissemination of innovative practice at scientific meetings and publications	Annual conference Regional meetings Peer-reviewed journal Website
Association for Medical Education in Europe (AMEE) Simulation Special Interest Group http://www.mededworld.org/SIGs.aspx A European association of medical and health professional educators with a special interest group in simulation Number of members: invited members only during establishment phase	• Promote simulation in the broadest sense • The SIG intends to work within the AMEE community • Promote opportunities for relationship with other professional associations, such as the different societies for simulation • Bridge the gap between educationalist and the simulation communities and between the different professions • Facilitate simulation as an educational method • Networking between countries in order to learn from others and move away from locally adapted practices to evidence based practice	AMEE meetings Separate expert group meeting Open meeting during AMEE congress
Turkish Association for Medical Education in Europe SP Special Interest Group Number of members :15	• Promote SP methodology in health sciences education • Exchange and promote the use of simulation within Turkish medical education	Regional annual meeting

Other international associations include the Society in Europe for Simulation Applied to Medicine (SESAM) and the UK-based Association for Simulated Practice in Healthcare (ASPiH). These organizations have similar goals and are defined largely by their geographical boundaries with all the incumbent cultural differences. Both have an annual conference and ASPiH is launching a peer-reviewed journal and at their 2013 conference featured a keynote presentation on SP methodology. At a national level, the Australian Society for Simulation in Healthcare (ASSH) has a small special interest group in SP methodology. Regionally, the Ontario Simulation Network facilitates the development of SP practices in Canada.

Simulation-specific communities have a contemporary focus on the certification of individuals and the accreditation of centres and programmes. These areas of interest intersect with those of SP-focused associations. The ASPE is working with SSH to establish standards relevant to all simulation practitioners. Other areas of interest include clarification of terms, identification of effective practices, sharing of resources, establishing research priorities and facilitating their implementation – all the dimensions relevant for communities of practice.

Medical and health professions education communities

Some medical education professional communities have special interest groups for those working with in simulation. For example, the Association for Medical Education in Europe (AMEE) now has a special interest group in 'simulation'. Although this is a broader base of simulation practitioners, it has some advantages in bringing together simulation practitioners with experience and expertise in different modalities. Again, AMEE has an affiliation with ASPE, enabling targeted workshop activities at their annual conference. At a national level, the Turkish Association for Medical Education in Europe hosts a special interest group in SP methodology.

Profession and specialty specific simulation communities

There are profession-specific simulation communities such as the International Nursing Association for Clinical Simulation and Learning (INACSL). The association promotes research and disseminates evidence-based practice standards for clinical simulation methodologies and learning environments. Although SP methodology is not its core focus, there is evidence that the method is valued alongside other simulation modalities. The International Pediatric Simulation Society (IPSS) promotes and supports multidisciplinary simulation education, training and research with a focus on neonates, children and adolescents. Although its focus has largely been associated with manikin-based immersive simulations and the use of task trainers, recent meetings have seen the emergence of SPs and simulated parents as important simulation modalities.

Healthcare communication communities

Given the critical nature of SPs in the development of clinical communication skills, professional communities with these skills at their core also support SP practitioners. Examples include the European Association for Communication in Healthcare (EACH) and the American Academy on Communication in Healthcare (AACH). Both associations offer resources to members on how to work effectively with SPs in teaching and assessing clinical communication skills, host an annual joint conference, a journal, other publications and a range of courses including residential intensives that help to build networks.

Conclusion

In this chapter, we have focused attention on SP practitioners rather than SPs themselves. We have considered the breadth and depth of their responsibilities and how these are determined locally. We have considered factors important for the development of SP practitioners, especially those offered by professional associations, networks and societies, each with overlapping but nuanced differences by simulation modality, geographical region or discipline. The professional communities cited here were started by pioneers in healthcare simulation and appear to have made a significant difference to the development of

simulation practices. The founders of these associations are largely all still practising, indicative of the relative recency of the professionalization of healthcare simulation practitioners. However, for SP practitioners, the career pathway remains unclear and perhaps this adds richness to their practice. We have noted the challenge of developing a new identity (as an SP practitioner) as it sits alongside or becomes the dominant role for the practitioner. It is obviously important that SP practitioners work closely with SPs in shaping SP practices. Viewing the roles of professional communities through a theoretical lens of communities of practice has helped to focus on the ways in which SP practitioners are supported in the development of SP methodology. It is apparent that professional communities play a critical role in the development of SP practitioners by providing opportunities for them to participate in meaningful activities and have facilitated sharing of resources and experiences.

References

1 Lave J and Wenger E (1991) *Situated Learning: Legitimate Peripheral Participation*. Cambridge University Press, Cambridge.
2 Wenger E (1998) *Communities of Practice: Learning, Meaning and Identity*. Cambridge University Press, Cambridge.
3 Morris C (2012) Reimaging the 'firm': clinical attachments as time sepnt in communities of practice. In: Cook V, Daly C and Newman M (eds) *Work-Based Learning in Clinical Settings*, pp. 11–25. Radcliffe Publishing, London.
4 Nestel D, Pritchard S, Blackstock F, Keating J and Bowman K (2013) Simulated patient methodology across three continents: a qualitative interview-based study. Presented at AMEE 2013, Prague, Association for Medical Education in Europe.
5 Gaba D (2007) The future vision of simulation in healthcare. *Simulation in Healthcare*, **2**: 126–35.
6 McGaghie WC, Issenberg SB, Petrusa ER and Scalese RJ (2010) A critical review of simulation-based medical education research: 2003–2009. *Medical Educattion*, **44**(1): 50–63.

Part 2
Theoretical Perspectives

5 Learning theories and simulated patient methodology

Margaret Bearman and Debra Nestel
Monash University, Clayton, Australia

KEY MESSAGES

- Simulated patient (SP) methodology has affective or emotional dimensions and learning theories should consider this important aspect of learning with SPs.
- *Cognitive load theory* and *scaffolding* provide theoretical rationales to support the design of SP methodology.
- *Narrative learning theory* offers ways to support *reflective practice*. It permits the learner to situate their reflections within the broader story of their learning; it provides an understanding of the various points of view within an SP encounter.
- *Threshold concepts* are 'akin to a portal, opening up a new and previously inaccessible way of thinking about something'(1). 'Patient-centred care' may act as a threshold concept and SP encounters may help learners access new ways of thinking and practising.

OVERVIEW

This chapter explores a range of learning theories which inform SP methodology. It outlines three different ways of theorizing about learning, which provide insights into the unique educational opportunities afforded by SP methodology. Cognitive load theory and scaffolding are introduced as ways of thinking about the SP-based curriculum. Reflective practice and narrative learning concepts are applied to manage some of the key learnings which emerge from a learner–SP encounter. Finally, threshold concepts are presented, as a way of understanding the possible transformative power of SP methodology with respect to patient-centred care.

Introduction

This chapter focuses on learning theories that inform SP methodology. The definition of learning or educational theory is in itself somewhat amorphous. Here we take the view that a learning theory is a conceptual framework that assists teachers in understanding how learners develop in comprehension, skills, attitudes and performances. Simulation as an overall methodology is well supported by a range of these theories(2,3). The most prominent of these relate to experiential learning, in particular as introduced by Kolb(4). This is outlined in Chapter 3, where Kolb's experiential learning cycle is discussed with specific reference to simulation design. In brief, Kolb's learning theory, emphasizes the concrete experience – the *doing* – and the reflective component – the *thinking* through a cycle of reflecting, conceptualizing and planning. This chapter expands upon some of the concepts relevant to Kolb's cycle but also highlights other approaches to understanding how learners benefit from SP methodology.

Simulated Patient Methodology: Theory, Evidence and Practice, First Edition. Edited by Debra Nestel and Margaret Bearman.
© 2015 John Wiley & Sons, Ltd. Published 2015 by John Wiley & Sons, Ltd.

Educational theories are just one type of theory that has application to SP methodology. Other chapters in this book expand upon alternative theoretical perspectives. In Chapter 6, Smith *et al.* examine the dramatic arts, with a focus on supporting SPs in their performance. Murtagh presents the sociological perspective in understanding the benefits and limitations of authenticity in SP encounters in Chapter 7, and McNaughton and Hodges contextualize SP methodology against the competing and constructing discourses of health professional education in Chapter 8.

One of the features of learning theories is their rather overwhelming diversity. Rather than attempting to be comprehensive, we outline three approaches that have particular insights into SP methodology. The purpose is to present theory in a way that can assist educators and SPs alike in understanding how to optimize the learning interaction which forms the core of SP methodology. These are not *recipes* for learning but different ways of understanding how healthcare professionals and students (learners) can develop their practice as a consequence of working with SPs. We believe that a key feature of SP work is the development of the emotional or affective dimension of learning. The approaches presented here all touch on the notion of working within a practice, which, by its nature, requires learners to manage intimate interpersonal situations.

The first set of theories concern supporting the learner and are most relevant to the design of simulation activities. *Cognitive load theory* is an empirical theory, with its roots in neuropsychology, and has broad application to most human cognition. On the other hand, *scaffolding* is strongly associated with education and, while its empirical roots are in child development, its approach in higher education is more conceptually driven. Together, these theories provide insight into how the design of SP encounters can enhance learning. The second approach concerns the learning process itself. Key educational concepts such as *constructivism* and *reflective practice* are explored. These provide insight into how learners come to develop consciously their practice as a consequence of working with SPs. *Narrative learning* is introduced to assist educators in framing some of the complexities of SP methodology. The final approach considers how SP methodology is ideally matched to teaching patient-centred care,

through the notion of *threshold concepts*. Threshold concepts are a way of understanding the seismic shifts that happen to a learner, fundamentally altering how they understand and approach their practice.

Supporting the learner: *cognitive load theory* and *scaffolding*

Cognitive load theory is an empirical learning theory that proposes ways to structure teaching in order to optimize learning. The core of cognitive load theory states that a learner's working memory, or the part of consciousness that can process information, has significant limitations. Van Merriënboer and Sweller(5) noted that working memory allows a learner's mind to 'actively process no more than two to four elements simultaneously. It is able to deal with information for no more than a few seconds and almost all information is lost after about 20 seconds unless it is refreshed by rehearsal'. To use an analogy, working memory forms a bottleneck to learning, as most of the reasoning and performance cognitive power lie in long-term memory(6). If a learner is overwhelmed, they will have difficulty in processing the learning from the simulated environment and may simply not remember what has occurred(7). The essential design principle is to reduce the extraneous cognitive load that does not assist with learning and to amplify opportunities to engage with the learning aspects of the task(6). In SP methodology, a key issue is that the form of the examination or the simulated encounter is not overly complex, as this will add to the extraneous load on the learner. Just as importantly, educators should be mindful of the effect that emotions have on the learners' capacity to process new information: in simulation emotions can overwhelm learning(7). This is not to say that SP encounters should always be predictable and avoid important affective learning, as this is the methodology's strength. However, it is worth ensuring that learners already have reasonable skills or experience in interpersonal communication before exposing them to difficult emotional situations.

One of the instructional design techniques that complements cognitive load theory is *scaffolding*. Scaffolding is a term that has been used since the 1970s and it has come to refer to the way in which learners are supported, such as through constraining the number of factors within a task or focusing the attention of a learner on a task or allowing learners to model advanced performance(8). A key factor is the slow removal of the *scaffold* supports, which ultimately allows the learner to perform independently at a more advanced rate(8). Scaffolding can be used to manage learners' challenges with the limitations of their working memory. Learners may commence with simple interactions and then progress to more complex and generally more authentic interactions. For example, in a breaking bad news scenario, novices can be refocused and guided by the SP, but as the student skill and confidence progress, the SP may provide fewer *cues*. Additionally or simultaneously, novices can be presented with an emotionally neutral case, before being introduced to cases that have significant affective impact.

Making sense of the SP encounter: reflective practice, constructivism and narrative learning

As Kolb's learning cycle indicates, much of the learning when working with SP methodology occurs when the learner makes sense of the simulated experience and develops new understandings, skills and practices as a consequence. *Reflective practice* is one type of educational approach that is associated with this development process(9). Of particular note are the ideas of Donald Schön, whose work explored the way in which learning takes place through *reflection-in-action*, the thinking and adjustment that occur in the moment during the learning experience, and *reflection-on-action*, which occurs after the learning experience(10). This reflective process is mostly managed through the process of debriefing after an SP encounter. As outlined by Nestel *et al.* in Chapter 10, the debriefing processes that enable the learners to construct an understanding of the simulation experience are critical for enhancing learning through simulation methodologies(11).

Reflective practice is often considered to be aligned with *constructivism*, a paradigm where the learner is central to negotiating their own learning. The emphasis (and in fact onus) here is on the learner actively directing their own learning(12), in contrast to the traditional model which emphasizes the role of the teacher. One of the major critiques of reflective practice is that the goal becomes 'reflection itself at the expense of attaining actual knowledge and skills'(13). However, constructivist theory argues that the internal process of the learner must always contribute to learning. In other words, reflective practice is a necessary foundation for further development, although not perhaps the entire building. We would argue that SP methodology has significant advantages in integrating reflective practice with skill development, because the learner can rapidly and iteratively repeat the simulation, drawing directly on prior experience and feedback to adapt and develop their performance actively.

There are other concerns about reflective practice. Boud and Walker warn(9, p. 194): 'Because emotions and feelings are often downplayed in educational settings, it is common for reflection to be treated as if it were an intellectual exercise, a simple matter of thinking rigorously. However … emotions are central to all learning … One of the most common outcomes of intellectualizing reflection, is, ironically, that of leaving the student in disarray'. Reflection, both in group debriefing environments and later as an individual exercise, can be a highly emotive process in SP work. Learners can be overwhelmed by the reflective process unless the educator can provide some structures to help make sense of the experience.

One way to overcome this is to consider *narrative learning* theory as a framework for educators and for learners. Narrative learning draws from the notion that stories are key to any form of human learning(14), that we make sense of any form of encounter by understanding it as a story. 'Stories are powerful precisely because they engage learners at a deeply human level. Stories draw us into an experience at more than a cognitive level; they engage our spirit, our imagination, our heart and this engagement is complex and holistic'(15, p. 62). Critically, stories always are told from *perspectives*, they allow *points of view* that can accommodate conflicting accounts of an incident(16).

SP methodology permits multiple perspectives of the scenario *story* to be told: the SP, the simulated healthcare provider (learner), even the observers. Drawing from narrative theory, learners can be assisted in *making sense* of their simulated encounter by deliberately placing it within the context of broader stories or 'life narratives'. Learners may find it easier to comprehend the SP perspective as a narrative: this may be done by simply asking the SP to recount briefly the *story* of their experience. Learners can be asked to place the learning from the scenario in the overall narrative of their own professional development – what does this *story* change for the next encounter? Storytelling or *narrative learning* allows for the gap between the simulated and the real by thinking of the simulation encounter as a *story within a story*, a way of understanding a learning event within the overall life story of the learner.

As suggested, thinking about learning in terms of storytelling can help support the reflection phase of simulations, through providing tools for the learner post-debriefing. Writing reflective journals with structured activities can assist. For example: write the story of what happened within this encounter from the perspective of the physiotherapist; or, if you had to rewrite the story with a different ending, what would it look like? Narrative learning theory argues that the act of narrating or writing is itself the act of constructing learning(15).

New ways of understanding: threshold concepts

An alternative theoretical lens for the learning that takes place in SP encounters is that of *threshold concepts*, reported by Meyer and Land(1). They described a threshold concept as 'akin to a portal, opening up a new and previously inaccessible way of thinking about something. It represents a transformed way of understanding or interpreting or viewing something without which the learner cannot progress'. That is, a threshold concept can change the way one thinks about and practises something. With reference to SP methodology, we argue that thoughtfully designed SP-based educational activities can address the threshold concept of *patient-centred care*. Although patient-centred care is simple enough to describe, its enactment is clearly challenging, as evidenced by research that demonstrated that learners and professionals often lack empathic and other communication skills(17–20), and more generally by patient dissatisfaction with healthcare services related to compromised or absent patient-centred

care(21–24). SP-based encounters and feedback can change the way in which learners think about patient-centred care.

Health professional education is focused on developing learners to think as clinicians (rather than as patients). However, the experience of receiving healthcare as patients is completely different to the experience of giving healthcare as clinicians. Failing to understand the differences may impede the understanding and practice of patient-centred care. SPs are well placed to bridge this gap in supporting learners to appreciate patient perspectives. SPs can articulate how their ideas, concerns and expectations align or misalign with those of the simulated health professional. Otherwise, areas of complementarity may go unnoticed by learners (and therefore no learning occurs) and areas of tension may simply be ignored as the learner moves on to another challenge. Further, as learners progress through their professional education, they seek identification with clinicians (often as role models) rather than with patients. This is a normal process of professionalization but it may diminish their ability to grasp patient-centred care (depending on their choice of role model).

Meyer and Land argue that, 'as a consequence of comprehending a threshold concept there may thus be a transformed internal view of subject matter, subject landscape or even world view'(1). They describe the transformation as occurring in different time frames – from *sudden* to *protracted* – and that the transition can be *troublesome* for learners. Thinking about patient-centred care as a threshold concept reflects the ways in which many learners seem to experience their professional healthcare education. Reflecting on our experiences of working with many learners over many years with SPs, during debriefing with learners and SPs a 'light-bulb' moment often occurs as learners come to appreciate the value of patient perspectives in their ability to provide patient-centred and safe care. These light-bulb moments may destabilize the learner, leaving them with a sense of discomfort as the learner comes to accept a different way of thinking and practising(25).

Learners who do not grasp threshold concepts may be left in a state of *liminality*. This is described as 'a suspended state in which understanding approximates to a kind of mimicry or lack of authenticity'(1). Having witnessed an SP provide feedback to a learner on his attempt at making an empathic statement that seemed like 'empathy by numbers', the learner was confronted by the realization that simply *going through the motions of patient-centred communication* is insufficient – that the learner must move their internal view to one of genuinely valuing patient centredness. In another example, in a hybrid simulation in which the learner was excising a mole and closing the resulting wound, during the feedback the SP sought to understand why the learner had not picked up two cues during the simulation, one subtle ('I am really worried about this mole'), the other overt ('My sister died of malignant melanoma'). It was only on video review that the learner *heard* these statements. The learner had not been *really* listening to the SP during the simulation despite knowing about patient-centred care and thinking he was being patient-centred. He was unable to offer patient-centred care due to his complete attention focusing on the psychomotor skills of the procedural skill. The feedback was transformative, helping him to think in a new way about patient-centred care. It was salutary for all involved. SPs are in a powerful position to offer this illuminating feedback.

Conclusion

We have provided an overview of three theory-based approaches to learning. Although there are many others, we selected these because of their particular promise in helping to access the unique features of SP methodology. All three guide the design of SP learning activities and curricula. Thinking about SP methodology as *scaffolding*, the learner reduces the complexity of the task to *appropriate cognitive loads*, particularly affective load, which assists when focusing on the individual elements of SP activities. Thinking about *narrative learning theory* and *threshold concepts* can maximize the value of the total simulation experience, which is part and parcel of learning through SP encounters. All three approaches underpin the integrative role that SP methodology offers to learners, which helps them to assimilate and make connections in all facets of their work. It is very easy to fall into ritual or tokenistic forms of education, which emphasize that which learners are already expecting to hear(26), for example, the rehearsed history taking of name, date of birth and so on. Drawing

from theory can help SP methodology safeguard against tokenism, by promoting the value of the interactive, immersive and affective experience through which a learner can learn both to understand the patient perspective and to develop their own professional practice.

References

1 Meyer R and Land R (2003) *Threshold Concepts and Troublesome Knowledge: Linkages to Ways of Thinking and Practising Within the Disciplines*. Occasional Report 4, ETL Project, Universities of Edinburgh, Coventry and Durham.
2 Bearman M, Nestel D and Andreatta P (2013) Simulation-based medical education. In Walsh K (ed.) *Oxford Textbook of Medical Education*, pp. 186–97. Oxford University Press, Oxford.
3 Kaufman DM and Mann KV (2010) Teaching and learning in medical education: how theory can inform practice. In: Swanwick T (ed.) *Understanding Medical Education: Evidence, Theory and Practice*, pp. 16–36. Wiley-Blackwell, Oxford.
4 Kolb DA, Boyatzis RE and Mainemelis C (2001) Experiential learning theory: previous research and new directions. In: Sternberg RJ and Zhang L-F (eds) *Perspectives on Thinking, Learning and Cognitive Styles*, pp. 227–47. Lawrence Erlbaum Associates, Mahwah, NJ.
5 Van Merriënboer JJ and Sweller J (2010) Cognitive load theory in health professional education: design principles and strategies. *Medical Education*, **44**(1): 85–93.
6 Sweller J, Van Merrienboer JJ and Paas FGWC (1998) Cognitive architecture and instructional design. *Educational Psychology Review*, **10**(3): 251–96.
7 Fraser K, Ma I, Teteris E, Baxter H, Wright B and McLaughlin K (2012) Emotion, cognitive load and learning outcomes during simulation training. *Medical Education*, **46**(11): 1055–62.
8 Pea RD (2004) The social and technological dimensions of scaffolding and related theoretical concepts for learning, education and human activity. *Journal of the Learning Sciences*, **13**(3): 423–51.
9 Boud D and Walker D (1998) Promoting reflection in professional courses: the challenge of context. *Studies in Higher Education*, **23**(2): 191–206.
10 Schön DA (1987) *Educating the Reflective Practitioner*. Jossey-Bass, San Francisco.
11 Issenberg SB, McGaghie WC, Petrusa ER, Gordon DL and Scalese RJ (2005) Features and uses of high-fidelity medical simulations that lead to effective learning: a BEME systematic review. *Medical Teacher*, **27**(1), 10–28.
12 Biggs J (1996) Enhancing teaching through constructive alignment. *Higher Education*, **32**(3): 347–64.
13 Hodges B (2006) Medical education and the maintenance of incompetence. *Medical Teacher*, **28**(8): 690–6.

14 Bruner JS (1996) *The Culture of Education*: Harvard University Press.

15 Clark MC and Rossiter M (2008) Narrative learning in adulthood. In: Merriam SB (ed.) *Third Update on Adult Learning Theory. New Directions for Adult and Continuing Education, No. 119*, pp. 61–70. Jossey-Bass, San Francisco.

16 Charon R (2000). Reading, writing and doctoring: literature and medicine. *American Journal of the Medical Sciences*, **319**(5): 285–91.

17 Easter D and Beach W (2004) Competent patient care is dependent upon attending to empathic opportunities presented during interview sessions. *Current Surgery*, **61**(3): 313–8.

18 Levinson W, Gorawara-Bhat R and Lamb J (2000) A study of patient clues and physician responses in primary care and surgical settings. *JAMA*, **284**(8): 1021–7.

19 Roberts C, Wass V, Jones R, Sarangi S and Gillett A (2003) A discourse analysis study of 'good' and 'poor' communication in an OSCE: a proposed new framework for teaching students. *Medical Education*, **37**(3): 192–201.

20 Spiegel W, Zidek T, Maier M, Vutuc C, Isak K, Karlic H, *et al.* (2009) Breaking bad news to cancer patients: survey and analysis. *Psychooncology*, **18**(2): 179–86.

21 Richards N and Coulter A (2007) *Is the NHS Becoming More Patient-Centred? Trends from the National Surveys of NHS Patients in England 2002–07*. Picker Institute Europe, Oxford.

22 Gerteis M, Edgman-Levitan S, Daley J and Delbanco T (1993) *Through the Patient's Eyes: Understanding and Promoting Patient-Centered Care*. Jossey-Bass, San Francisco.

23 Darzi A (2008) *High Quality Care for All. NHS Next Stage Review Final Report*, CM 7432. Department of Health, London.

24 Aiken LH, Sermeus W, Van den Heede K, Sloane DM, Busse R, McKee M, *et al.* (2012) Patient safety, satisfaction and quality of hospital care: cross sectional surveys of nurses and patients in 12 countries in Europe and the United States. *BMJ*, **344**: e1717.

25 Cousin G (2006) An introduction to threshold concepts. *Planet*, (**17**): 4–5.

26 Bearman M and Ajjawi R (2013) Avoiding tokenism in health professional education. *Medical Education*, **47**(1): 9–11.

6 The dramatic arts and simulated patient methodology

Cathy M Smith[1], Tanya L Edlington[2], Richard Lawton[3] and Debra Nestel[4]

[1]University of Toronto, Toronto, Canada
[2]Melbourne, Victoria, Australia
[3]Ignite Coaching, Melbourne, Australia
[4]Monash University, Clayton, Australia

 KEY MESSAGES

- Dramatic arts theories and practices deepen our understanding of simulated patient (SP).
- Terms used in dramatic arts have been appropriated into SP methodology.
- Although there are similarities between SP and actor performances, there are also fundamental differences related to purpose – the centrality of the learner.
- Elements of SP performance informed by dramatic arts theories include creating character, enacting the narrative and relating to the audience.

OVERVIEW

SP methodology has adopted many terms from dramatic performance, such as actor, role, cast and script. This chapter explores these and other important concepts from the dramatic arts with the intention of deepening our understanding of SP practices. We draw on the work of theatre practitioners such as Stanislavski, Spolin, Boal and Brecht. SP performance elements informed by the dramatic arts include creating character, enacting the narrative and relating to the audience. Other theoretical concepts that have relevance to SP performance are explored, such as improvisation, textual information (major and minor units), mirror mechanisms and circles of attention.

Introduction

In this chapter, we explore the role of dramatic arts theories in SP methodology. An overview of theoretical conceptions of SPs and performance is provided. drawing on the work of Stanislavski, Spolin, Boal, Brecht and others to offer insights into elements of SP performance: creating character, enacting the narrative and relating to the audience.

Simulated patients and performance

Performance is a key component of SP methodology. SP encounters are described as being 'the most recognizable and productive use of performance in medical education'(1, p. 160). In the broadest sense, performance refers to 'the doing of an action'(2). Through the lens of the dramatic arts, performance can be thought

Simulated Patient Methodology: Theory, Evidence and Practice, First Edition. Edited by Debra Nestel and Margaret Bearman.
© 2015 John Wiley & Sons, Ltd. Published 2015 by John Wiley & Sons, Ltd.

of as representing behaviours associated with all human activity(3–5). In a narrower sense, performance can be defined as 'an individual performer's or group's rendering or interpretation of a work, part, role'(6). However, the notion of an observer or audience is implicit(3,7). SPs render or interpret patient roles, interacting with an audience of learners (both the learners in the scenario and the observers). This type of performance corresponds to that of an actor. As such, examining key acting theories and practices can deepen our understanding of contemporary SP practice.

The connection between dramatic arts and western medicine has existed since the time of the ancient Greeks(8). More recently, Hodges identified 'performance discourse' as a paradigm of competence, with SPs an integral element and dramatic arts a critical theoretical foundation(7). Performance and dramatic arts theories and techniques in the training of health professional learners are increasingly reported(1,9–25). Additionally, these approaches are being explored in the training of simulation practitioners(26) and for SPs(8,27–36).

SP performance is frequently described with terminology taken from the dramatic arts. SPs are often referred to as *actors*(8,32,35,37–40). *Cast* in a *role* written as a *script* or scenario containing *lines of dialogue, stage directions, intentions* and *objectives*, SPs are then *directed* or *coached* at *rehearsals* and *dry runs* where they are expected to be *off-book* in preparation for a performance with an *audience*, sometimes on a *stage* that has a *set* and *props*. They wear *makeup* and have a *wardrobe*. They stay *in character* unless they are asked to come *out of role*. After their performance, they *de-role*. The often unconscious co-opting of this language to name and frame SP performance has occurred because, in many ways, SP and actor performances are similar.

Simulated patient and actor performances

Central to any actor's performance is the creation of character. Their instruments are themselves: they simultaneously integrate domains (cognitive, physical, psychological), in order to pretend that they are someone else, for an audience(4). Although SPs also do this, they do something different from actors too, relating to the *purpose* of performance. The actor is an artist, bringing to life a character in the service of the playwright, a director's vision or a producer. SPs are 'patients' as teachers. They embody another person, such as a patient, not so much to pretend that they are this other but to serve as their proxy and to work towards supporting clinician learning. Ultimately, for SPs, it is always about the learner.

Acting and SP performance are distinctive genres, each with a specific *purpose* that in turn affects both the *form or* appearance and *style or* technique, of the performance. Within each genre, there are sub-genres, again related to the purpose, that create nuances in form and style. SP performance in a formative assessment with first-year students may be different from that in a summative assessment for licensure, just as an actor's stage performance in a Shakespearean tragedy would be different from that in a television sitcom.

This relationship between SP and actor performance is complicated and is only beginning to be investigated(8,28–31,34). Despite the many differences, there are also many similarities. Nelles, in an ethnographic account of her work as an SP, noted, 'While it can be said that we are not acting, it is also true that we are not *not* acting'(30, p. 56). There is much that can be drawn from dramatic arts theories and practice to inform, in a generalizable way, SP performance.

Elements of simulated patient performance

Creating character

Effective SP performance is rooted in the concept of realism, defined as a 'close resemblance to what is real; fidelity of representation, rendering the precise details of the real thing or scene'(41). SP performances must be authentic in terms of both clinical details and the human experience represented because SPs are proxies for real patients(8,37,38,42–45). SPs are trained to portray a role so that the learners believe that they are dealing with a real patient. In this way, learners are engaged and immersed as if they were in a real clinical encounter, ensuring that the experiential learning process is fully realized and connects meaningfully with real work(26,46). Challenges, however, can come with defining what a 'real' SP performance is as reality is subjective and complex – what is real to one person may be false to another.

Russian theatre practitioner Constantine Stanislavski (1863–1938) provides guidance for the creation of this type of realistic character. Considered the first modern acting teacher, he developed an evolving psychophysical 'system' of acting, where none had existed before, and in reaction to the often mannered and exaggerated performances that had characterized nineteenth century stage performance(4,47). He explored ways to help actors portray characters authentically. He sought 'truth on stage', which had much to do with the actor believing they were in the situation and behaving sincerely rather than just mimicking a surface reality(47). *Relaxation* and *concentration* were key skills(47).

Actors were required to determine the *given circumstances* of the play, the actual information contained in the text(47). In addition, actors also had to create the *sub-textual* information – the imagined life beneath the surface that was not spoken but manifested in non-verbal behaviours(48). This *sub-text* was created by determining the *given circumstances* and then using the *'magic if'*(47). The actor had to ask, 'If I was this character at this moment of the play, what would I do?' This process develops 'empathic imagination … a cognitive skill set that helps one to imagine the experiences and responses of another person'(1, p. 159).

Stanislavski also devised a complex analytical process for actors to negotiate moment-by-moment through a play. At its core, the text is divided into major and minor *units*. Although these divisions are linked to changes in the given circumstances of the text (e.g. new information, entrances or exits of other characters), they are also somewhat subjective. The smallest *units* are *objectives* (what the character wants), which are achieved through a series of *actions*. *Actions* are described using an active, infinitive, transitive verb (e.g. to confront her, to placate her, to woo her). Defining actions (related to specific objectives) allows them to be set, concretely done, repeated, changed and refined in an iterative manner as rehearsals progress(47). Through this analysis, each actor finds a unique way to portray a character.

In his later work, Stanislavski had his actors create and improvise a continuous sequence of *physical actions*, performed silently and 'motivated by an inner sense of truth and a belief in what the actor is doing'(47, p. 135). This is an active,

physical, experiential process designed to trigger and simultaneously connect thoughts, emotions and physicality. Stanislavski came to realize that actors should not deliberately summon their emotions because this could be harmful to them and, because emotions were not controllable or repeatable, this could result in erratic and often forced, false performances(32,47).

An emphasis on physicality has been a central feature of the work of many subsequent practitioners(49–52), leading to theories and practices of *embodied* performance. In this holistic body–mind approach, 'the actor uses his or her body to communicate meaning to an audience. This is accomplished by language, by nonverbal communication(nvc), and by mirror mechanisms that support empathy'(53, p. 186). *Non-verbal communication* includes elements such as facial expression, eye movement, gesture, posture, use of space, distance between individuals, tempo, rhythm and vocal gestures related to categories such as pitch, pace, enunciation and silence(53). *Mirror mechanisms* describes a process through which 'an observer mimics, resonates with or re-creates the mental life of others based on direct observation of their movements'(53, p. 132).

Aspects of Stanislavski's work and embodied performance can guide SPs in creating realistic characters. SP practitioners have used Stanislavskian techniques to help SPs create believable patients(8,32,34,54,55). A systematic approach, starting with careful analysis of the written information in a role, allows SPs to be clear about the *given circumstances*. Writing scenarios with clear *objectives* (such as a patient's expectations for the visit) helps SPs to stay grounded and focused. Encouraging SPs to develop their empathic imagination or 'compassion'(30, p. 60), by using techniques that include the *'magic if'* to explore the *sub-text* – the life that is just under the surface of the patient they are representing – imbues their portrayal with greater humanity. Guiding SPs to play doable *actions* (e.g. to challenge him, to plead with her, to negotiate with him) grounded in their *objectives* rather than expecting them to display heightened emotions on demand ensures repeatable, consistent performances that will evoke appropriate emotions in an unforced and naturalistic manner. Experimenting with *non-verbal communication* will help to trigger further nuances that cannot always be articulated through language and/or text. Using video recordings of real patients with SPs to explore *mirror mechanism* responses can add depth to their portrayals. These suggestions barely scratch the surface of the possibilities: how SPs embody emotion and affect is a dense, layered, often individualized process(34). As with actors, for safety, it is important to develop de-roling strategies for SPs, especially if the portrayal has been intense(27,30,55,56).

Enacting the narrative

SPs and learners co-create the narrative of a clinical encounter. SPs often work from a semi-scripted scenario. Learners are unscripted, although the broader definition of performance suggests that these learners are not naive and, in fact, are playing a role – themselves – in which they understand both the structure and expectations of their performance(1,26). For example, a consultation with a family doctor will have a different narrative structure than a visit to the pharmacist, reflecting the different scopes of practice. Gathering patient information requires a different approach from breaking bad news or performing a physical examination.

Although SPs usually have some specific information and scripted lines, they have to decide when and how to deliver this information. They often portray their role many times consecutively to learners who have very different approaches. They are also simultaneously in and out of role, internally observing and keeping track of the interaction in order to assess or provide feedback. This is an increased cognitive load and can affect their ability both to stay in role and then provide accurate assessment(57). In a summative assessment, SP behaviour has to be rigorously standardized, even though they are dealing with unstandardized learners, which puts even greater demand on them to negotiate through the narrative.

Principles of improvisational theatre can be helpful in guiding SPs through this uncertainty and ambiguity. Improvisation is broadly defined as a 'work … produced on the spur of the moment'(58). Although it is a technique that is used in many contexts to help actors explore the inner life of their characters (as Stanislavski did), improvisational theatre is a type of performance with many diverse styles. Viola Spolin (1906–1994) developed an experiential system of actor training called *Theatre Games*, based on a series of scaffolded

exercises that holistically explore the development of the senses, intuition, truth, spontaneity and connection to the environment and other actors(59).

Many diverse improvisational formats have developed(60–62). A key concept that emerged from this style of theatre relates to *agreement*. 'The first rule of improvisation is *agree*. Always *agree* and *say "yes"*. … The second rule of improvisation is not only to say *"yes"*, but *"yes and"'*(63, p. 84). '*Yes*' means that you are in relationship with your partner, accepting their *offer*, rather *blocking* or trying to control a situation. '*And*' means you are taking responsibility for moving the action forward and offering creative opportunities to your partner(64). Even though improvisational theatre appears to be of-the-moment, it has a strong structural container. Rehearsal, involving practice and drills of particular games and exercises and feedback, solidifies the development of an improviser's skills.

These principles provide guidance for SPs in negotiating the narrative. Making sure roles contain details relevant to the particular narrative format of the scenario provides the context that SPs need to give assured performances. Having protocols for dealing with unexpected questions or situations or how much and when to give information can be helpful so that SPs do not break character. Rehearsing SPs with various types of anticipated learner performances provides benchmarking so they gain a sense of how to tell their story effectively. Having SPs play learners in rehearsals can also help them to discover unanticipated aspects of the role and can promote empathic understanding of the learner's task. Creating exercises that build skills by deconstructing aspects of a patient role (e.g. physical affect, saying an opening line in different ways, imaging a typical day for this person) and then integrating these discoveries back into the role can help develop fluidity, depth and dimensionality in role portrayal.

The rules of '*agree*' and '*yes and*' apply as long as this serves the learning objectives of the scenario. The essence is that SPs will co-create with learners rather than block them by shutting down (e.g. breaking out of role or getting flustered). The potential benefits of building improvisational techniques into SP practice may alleviate the increased cognitive load related to role portrayal and subsequent feedback and assessment(57).

Relating to the audience

SPs navigate numerous boundaries while interacting with their audience of learners. While performing, they are in role and out of role – embodying a realistic patient, while monitoring what both they and the learner are doing, in order to deliver prompts or key information or to demonstrate a particular affect in response to a learner's cue. A *time-out* might be called where SPs have to neutralize their presence as a discussion occurs between facilitator and learner. The SP may be required to resume at the very point the time-out was called – no matter how intense the moment – or go backwards in the interaction, even starting it again(42,65). The simulation may be in front of a large group of learners in a theatre setting, interacting with one learner in a *fish bowl* or with multiple learners, one after the other, in a *round-robin* exercise. When the simulation ends, SPs come out of role to give feedback or to assess the learner. SPs may do this many times in a session. Negotiating these tasks demands concentration, focus and stamina from SPs so that they are always aware of where they are within the simulation in relation to the learner(s).

Circles of attention, as defined by Stanislavski, help actors focus on their relationship with an audience and each other. The *small circle* includes an actor's internal space and the closely surrounding external space. The *medium circle* is the space between two or more actors. Finally, there is the *large circle*, which includes extended gestures, the whole audience and the larger performance space(47). Another boundary concept is the *fourth wall*, 'an imaginary barrier that separates the performers on stage from the audience'(66). It can help actors concentrate, create greater intimacy on-stage and increase the realism of the theatrical illusion for the audience(29). Berthold Brecht (1898–1956) had his actors break the *fourth wall* by directly addressing the audience, in an effort to confront and inspire them to analyse what was happening rather than to escape into the illusion(67). Augusto Boal (1931–2009), in the Theatre of the Oppressed, dissolved the *fourth wall*, with audiences becoming active participants in the performance. A short scene illustrating a problem, related to complex issues such as social inequity, is played out by trained actors. A '*joker*' (facilitator) oversees the action, watched by the '*spec-actors*' (spectators), who at any point can stop the action, make suggestions about how to proceed or jump in to interact, taking the place of one of the actors and co-creating with them multiple new, hopefully more positive, outcomes that can be transferred to daily life(68).

Alraek and Baerheim explored how *circles of attention* provide structure for SPs as they adapt to a constantly shifting relationship with their audience(28). The *small circle* can help SPs access the patient's inner world or remove themselves energetically from learners during a time-out. The *medium circle* can be seen as the space helping the SP to stay connected with the learner. Being in this circle can remind SPs that they do not need to project their voice or physical gestures as they are often working in intimate spaces(30). The *large circle* includes the entire space in which the simulation is taking place, and also others in the space (e.g. learners, observers, clinicians, facilitators). Moving into this circle can help SPs to mark for themselves that they are stepping out of role and connecting with the audience and to give feedback. Jacobsen *et al.* noted that the concept of the *fourth wall* can be a useful tool for framing the relationship between the audience and performers in SP interactions(29). During small-group teaching, for example, the SP is behind the *fourth wall* with the learner. This wall gets broken when a facilitator calls a time-out to reflect with the learner. The wall shifts away from the SP (who is now outside the performance space) to encompass the learner, facilitator and other observers, then the wall shifts back to its initial position when the action resumes. When the SP comes out of role to give feedback to the learner, the *fourth wall* breaks in a Brechtian manner as the SP directly addresses the audience. *The fourth wall* might also dissolve, as envisioned by Boal, if the SP is asked to be in role with a consecutive series of learners, who each come up and try portions of the interview or who make suggestions from the audience in order to co-create diverse outcomes. Developing strategies so that SPs can recognize and negotiate the boundaries between themselves and learners also creates trust and provides safety for all involved in the simulation.

Conclusion

Exploring similarities and differences between acting and SP practice creates a deeper understanding of how to articulate key elements of and a language specific to SP performance. Although the dramatic arts traditions presented here are important, they are a small selection and culturally biased. The memorization of the facts contained in an SP role is just one of the many starting points for an SP portrayal. Consciously applied strategies based on established dramatic arts theories and practices, to embody realistic characters, confidently enact the narrative with learners and relate to their audience, help SPs strengthen the integrity of the process and increase their potential to engage learners in mindful, sincere encounters. Moreover, these strategies can inform performance practices in other simulation modalities.

References

1 Case GA and Brauner DJ (2010) Perspective: the doctor as performer: a proposal for change based on a performance studies paradigm. *Academic Medicine*, **85**(1): 159–63.
2 *Oxford English Dictionary* [Internet] (2013) Sep. Performance, n. 1a. Oxford University Press, Oxford.
3 Carlson M (1996) *Performance: a Critical Introduction*. Routledge, New York.
4 Gordon R (2006) *The Purpose of Playing: Modern Acting Theories in Perspective*. University of Michigan Press, Ann Arbor, MI.
5 Schechner R (2006) *Performance Studies: an Introduction*, 2nd edn. Routledge, New York.
6 *Oxford English Dictionary* [Internet] (2013) Sep. Performance, n. 4c. Oxford University Press, Oxford.
7 Hodges B. 2012 The shifting discourses of competence. In: Hodges B and Lingard L (eds) *The Question of Competence: Reconsidering Medical Education in the Twenty-First Century*, pp. 14–41. Cornell University Press, Ithaca, NY.
8 Wallace P (2007) *Coaching Standardized Patients: for Use in the Assessment of Clinical Competence*. Springer, New York.
9 Bourke LF (1991) The use of theatre in dental health education. *Australian Dental Journal*, **36**(4): 310–1.
10 Ball S (1993) Theatre in health education. In: Jackson T (ed.) *Learning Through Theatre: New Perspectives on Theatre in Education*, 2nd edn, pp. 227–38. Routledge, New York.
11 Brown KH and Gillespie D (1997) "We become brave by doing brave acts": teaching moral courage through the theater of the oppressed. *Literature and Medicine*, **16**(1): 108–20.
12 Shapiro J and Hunt L (2003) All the world's a stage: the use of theatrical performance in medical education. *Medical Education*, **37**(10): 922–7.
13 Wasylko Y and Stickley T (2003) Theatre and pedagogy: using drama in mental health nurse education. *Nurse Education Today*, **23**(6): 443–8.
14 Baerheim A and Alraek T (2005) Utilizing theatrical tools in consultation training. A way to facilitate students' reflection on action? *Medical Teacher*, **27**: 652–4.
15 Krüger C, Blitz-Lindeque JJ, Pickworth GE, Munro AJ and Lotriet M (2005) Communication skills for medical/dental students at the University of Pretoria: lessons learnt from a two-year study using a forum theatre method. *South African Family Practice*, **47**(6): 60–5.
16 Case GA and Micco G (2006) Moral imagination takes the stage: readers' theater in a medical context. *Journal for Learning Through the Arts*, **2**(1).
17 Dow AW, Leong D, Anderson A, Wenzel RP, Gennings C, Rodgers J, *et al.* (2007) Using theater to teach clinical empathy: a pilot study. *Journal of General Internal Medicine*, **22**(8): 1114–8.
18 Hoffman A, Utley B and Ciccarone D (2008) Improving medical student communication skills through improvisational theatre. *Medical Education*, **42**(5): 537–8.
19 Csörsz I, Molnar P and Csabai M (2011) Medical students on the stage: an experimental performative method for the development of relational skills. *Medical Teacher*, **33**(9): e489–94.
20 De la Croix A, Rose C, Wildig E and Willson S (2011) Arts-based learning in medical education: the students' perspective. *Medical Education*, **45**(11): 1090–100.
21 Hammer RR, Rian JD, Gregory JK, Bostwick JM, Birk CB, Chalfant L, *et al.* (2011) Telling the patient's story: using theatre training to improve case presentation skills. *Medical Humanities*, **37**(1): 18–22.
22 Kohn M (2011) Performing medicine: the role of theatre in medical education. *Medical Humanities*, **37**(1): 3–4.
23 Brett-Maclean P, Yiu V and Farooq A (2012) Exploring professionalism in undergraduate medical and dental education through forum theatre. *Journal for Learning Through the Arts*, **8**(1).
24 Love KI (2012) Using Theater of the Oppressed in nursing education: Rehearsing to be change agents. *Journal for Learning Through the Arts*, **8**(1).
25 Salam T, Collins M and Baker AM (2012) All the world's a stage: integrating theater and medicine for interprofessional team building in physician and nurse residency programs. *The Ochsner Journal*, **12**(4): 359–62.
26 Sanko JS, Shekhter I, Kyle RR, Di Benedetto S and Birnbach DJ (2013) Establishing a convention for acting in healthcare simulation: merging art and science. *Simulation in Heathcare*, **8**(4): 215–20.
27 McNaughton N, Tiberius R and Hodges B (1999) Effects of portraying psychologically and emotionally complex standardized patient roles. *Teaching and Learning in Medicine*, **11**(3): 135–41.
28 Alraek T and Baerheim A (2005) Elements from theatre art as learning tools in medical education. *Research in Drama Education*, **1**: 5–14.
29 Jacobsen T, Baerheim A, Lepp M and Schei E (2006) Analysis of role-play in medical communication training using a theatrical device the fourth wall. *BMC Medical Education*, **6**(1): 51.

30 Nelles LJ (2011) My Body, Their Story: Performing Medicine. *Canadian Theatre Review*, **146**(1): 55–60.

31 Taylor JS (2011) The moral aesthetics of simulated suffering in standardized patient performances. *Culture, Medicine, and Psychiatry*, **35**(2): 134–62.

32 Keltner NL, Grant JS and McLernon D (2011) Use of actors as standardized psychiatric patients facilitating success in simulation experiences. *Journal of Psychosocial Nursing and Mental Health Services*, **49**(5): 34–40.

33 Gormley G, Sterling M, Menary A and McKeown G (2012) Keeping it real! Enhancing realism in standardised patient OSCE stations. *The Clinical Teacher*, **9**(6): 382–6.

34 McNaughton NL (2012) A theoretical analysis of the field of human simulation and the role of emotion and affect in the work of standardized patients. Dissertation, University of Toronto.

35 Webster D, Seldomridge L and Rockelli L (2012) Making it real: using standardized patients to bring case studies to life. *Journal of Psychosocial Nursing and Mental Health Services*, **50**(5): 36–41.

36 Nestel D, Burn CL, Pritchard SA, Glastonbury R and Tabak D (2011) The use of simulated patients in medical education: Guide Supplement 42.1 Viewpoint. *Medical Teacher*, **33**(12): 1027–9.

37 Austin Z, Gregory P and Tabak D (2006) Simulated patients vs. standardized patients in objective structured clinical examinations. *American Journal of Pharmaceutical Education*, **70**(5): 119.

38 Kneebone R, Nestel D, Wetzel C, Black S, Jacklin R, Aggarwal R, *et al.* (2006) The human face of simulation: patient-focused simulation training. *Academic Medicine*, **81**(10): 919–24.

39 Nestel DF, Black SA, Kneebone RL, Wetzel CM, Thomas P, Wolfe JHN, *et al.* (2008) Simulated anaesthetists in high fidelity simulations for surgical training: feasibility of a training programme for actors. *Medical Teacher*, **30**(4): 407–13.

40 Kneebone RL (2009) Practice, rehearsal and performance: an approach for simulation-based surgical and procedure training. *JAMA*, **302**(12): 1336–8.

41 *Oxford English Dictionary* [Internet] (2013) Sep. Realism, n. 4a. Oxford University Press, Oxford.

42 Barrows HS (1993) An overview of the uses of standardized patients for teaching and evaluating clinical skills. *AAMC. Academic Medicine*, **68**(6): 443–51.

43 Nestel D, Cecchini M, Calandrini M, Chang L, Dutta R, Tierney T, *et al.* (2008) Real patient involvement in role development: evaluating patient focused resources for clinical procedural skills. *Medical Teacher*, **30**(5): 534–6.

44 Cleland JA, Abe K and Rethans JJ (2009) The use of simulated patients in medical education: AMEE Guide No. 42.1. *Medical Teacher*, **31**(6): 477–86.

45 Nestel D and Kneebone R (2010) Perspective: authentic patient perspectives in simulations for procedural and surgical skills. *Academic Medicine*, **85**(5): 889–93.

46 Dieckmann P, Manser T, Wehner T and Rall M (2007) Reality and fiction cues in medical patient simulation: an interview study with anesthesiologists. *Journal of Cognitive Engineering and Decision Making*, **1**(2): 148–68.

47 Stanislavski C (1984) *My Life in Art*. Geoffrey Bliss. London.

48 Stanislavski C (1972) *Building a Character*. Theatre Arts Books, New York.

49 Chekhov M (1953) *To the Actor: on the Technique of Acting*. Harper and Row, New York.

50 Artaud A (1958) *The Theater and Its Double*. Grove Press, New York.

51 Grotowski J (1968) *Towards a Poor Theater*. Simon and Shuster, New York.

52 Lecoq J (2001) *The Moving Body*. Routledge, New York.

53 Kemp R (2010) Embodied acting: cognitive foundations of performance. Dissertation, University of Pittsburgh.

54 Barrows HS (1987) *Simulated (Standardized) Patients and Other Human Simulations*. Health Sciences Consortium, Chapel Hill, NC.

55 McNaughton N, Ravitz P, Wadell A and Hodges BD (2008) Psychiatric education and simulation: a review of the literature. *Canadian Journal of Psychiatry*, **53**(2): 85–93.

56 Smith C (2012) Debriefing SPs after simulation events. www.vspn.edu.au (accessed 13 September 2013).

57 Newlin-Canzone ET, Scerbo MW, Gliva-Mcconvey G and Wallace AM (2013) The cognitive demands of standardized patients: understanding limitations in attention and working memory with the decoding of nonverbal behavior during improvisations. *Simulation in Heathcare*, **8**(4): 207–14.

58 *Oxford English Dictionary* [Internet] (2013) Sep. Improvisation, n. 2. Oxford University Press, Oxford.

59 Spolin V (1983) *Improvisation for the Theater*, 2nd edn. Northwestern University Press, Evanston, IL.

60 Salas J (1993) *Improvising Real Life: Personal Story in Playback Theatre*. Tusitala Publishing, New Paltz, NY.

61 Halpern C, Close D and Johnson K (1994) *Truth in Comedy: the Manual for Improvisation*. Meriwether, Colorado Springs, CO.

62 Johnstone K (2013) *Impro: Improvisation and the Theatre*. Routledge, New York.

63 Fey T (2011) *Bossypants*. Sphere, London and Regan Arthur Books/Little, Brown and Company, New York.

64 Madson PR (2005) *Improv Wisdom: Don't Prepare, Just Show Up*. Bell Tower, New York.

65 Wallace P (1997) Following the threads of an innovation: the history of standardized patients in medical education. *Caduceus*, **13**(2): 5–28.

66 Chandler D and Munday R (2011) *A Dictionary of Media and Communication*, Fourth wall. Oxford University Press, Oxford.

67 Brecht B (1949) A new technique of acting. *Theatre Arts*, **31**(1): 38–49.

68 Boal A (1992) *Games for Actors and Non-Actors*, 2nd edn. Routledge, London.

7 Simulated interaction and authentic interaction – a place for Conversation Analysis?

Ged M Murtagh

Imperial College London, London, UK

KEY MESSAGES

- Authentic interaction should be one of the primary goals of a simulated encounter.
- The degree of authenticity of the interaction between the simulated patient (SP) and learner is a key factor in shaping the acquisition of patient-centred communication skills.

- The simulated portrayal of 'real' patient stories can sometimes result in a power differential between the SP and learner, with the former taking a more inauthentic dominant role in the interaction.
- *Conversation Analysis* research could help ensure authentic communication behaviours by providing a firmer foundation for skills acquisition.

OVERVIEW

Authentic interaction is one of the primary goals when a SP is interacting with a medical learner. This chapter examines the issue of authenticity of interaction and considers how far sociological theory could contribute to informing the role of the SP. The chapter examines research on the socio-linguistic aspects of the SP–medical student encounter and proposes an alternative way of constructing SP roles.

Introduction

SPs have, for some time now, been an integral part of medical education and evidence suggests that SPs are effective in the teaching and assessment of professional skills(1). As an educational tool SP's can be used to emulate a patient who has come to the healthcare setting with a particular medical problem. The learner approaches the SP just as they would a real patient and attempts to deal with them competently by invoking appropriate communication skills. Normally the SP will come to the encounter with a patient role typically based on an interpretation of a real patient's story. The role may have certain character traits that will influence to a great extent how the SP interacts with the learner. The learner, on the other hand, receives a brief describing the patient and the problem they are presenting with, moments before entering the room to interview the patient. The learner is then presented with the challenge of accurately taking the patient's history in a way appropriate to the presenting problem and the patient's perspective. Encounters like this provide an effective forum for modelling examples of optimal/dysfunctional practice (opening these for scrutiny and discussion) and for identifying the characteristics of excellence.

The effectiveness of this forum is heavily contingent on what transpires between the two parties.

Simulated Patient Methodology: Theory, Evidence and Practice, First Edition. Edited by Debra Nestel and Margaret Bearman.
© 2015 John Wiley & Sons, Ltd. Published 2015 by John Wiley & Sons, Ltd.

If, for example, the SP's style of interaction is less authentic in some ways, this can negatively impact on the learning process. Much rests, therefore, on the communication behaviours that the SP enacts within the role. However, the way in which SPs actually interact in these encounters has, until recently, received little attention, which in itself raises a concern. The argument presented in this chapter is that, in the same way that high-fidelity simulated events will use and model features of actual clinical practice to ensure authenticity, the SP–learner encounter should incorporate methods that will capture key features of patients' actual communication behaviours in order to design a higher level of authenticity into the SP role.

Appearance and reality: the authenticity of interaction

Careful contextualization of learning and practice is critical in ensuring authenticity and a close relation between the actual and the simulated situation in which competence is being tested(1). There are, however, two potential barriers that may render this close relation, between the actual and simulated situation, problematic. The first is the use of real patients' accounts to construct SP roles. The rationale behind this is to ensure that real perspectives are incorporated into the process. However, the use of real patients' accounts' may not be enough to ensure authenticity from the point of view of the interaction process. The information supplied by the real patient to construct the role is, by its very nature, a second-hand account of what actually happened. Even the most accurate second-hand account will have difficulty escaping linguistic embellishment, a re-prioritization of events and the like, all of which are unintended consequences of designing roles in this way.

This leads to a consideration of the second potential barrier, which is that in an important sense the SP–learner encounter is almost the reverse of what may happen in real life. In reality, medical professionals typically have a '*mental map*' of the consultation whereas patients often do not know what to expect. In the simulated encounter, the SP, often having performed this role many times before, will arrive with the '*script*' and will, as a consequence, have a clearer idea or '*mental map*' of what will take place. The learner, on the other hand, who may be doing this for the first time, will go in with the brief which in many cases, for pedagogical reasons, does not always indicate what the learner should expect in any specific terms. Looked at in this light, it could be argued that the SP–learner encounter may actually run contra to what goes on when a doctor and patient meet. As a consequence of these two factors the SP may take a more (inauthentic) dominant role in the encounter, a role patients rarely take in real life.

This was one of the main findings of de la Croix and Skelton's study(2), which examined 100 videotaped assessed consultations between SPs and medical learners. de la Croix and Skelton extend the notion of professional dominance originating in Friedson's work(3) to examine interactional dominance evident through internal measures, such as talk time and interruptions. Examining the distribution of words and interruptions in SP encounters, de le Croix and Skelton discovered that SPs interrupted learners more frequently and as a consequence assumed a more dominant role within the encounter, something, they argue, is less likely to be found in real doctor–patient interaction. de la Croix and Skelton suggest educators should not lose sight of the difficulty of teaching general communication skills for the purposes of particular consultation scenarios. Otherwise, inauthentic interaction may result in the educational aims of the simulated encounter outweighing the overarching professional aims.

Although de la Croix and Skelton acknowledged the difficulty in defining what constitutes an interruption and also the simplicity of their analysis (counting words and interruptions as indicators of interactional dominance). The notion of interactional dominance that informs their analysis is not without its difficulties. The extent to which one party to an interaction is '*conversationally dominant*' over the other is a matter to be decided by the interlocutors themselves in real time as opposed to glossing sequences of talk as indices of conversational dominance after the event. Moreover, that doctors, for example, may talk more in the consultation tells us nothing about the substantive and dynamic nature of the talk itself. Patients often produce minimal responses to doctors' questions (irrespective of their design), which can place the onus back on the doctor to produce more talk(4,5). Even when the doctor actively seeks ways to engage and involve the patient more, the patient's actual verbal contribution to the consultation can remain relatively low compared with that of the doctor(6). To some extent, de la Croix and Skelton acknowledge these points. However, just as patients often naturally orient to taking the lead from the doctor, so learners in SP scenarios often orient to the fact that the SP may well take the lead. Irrespective of the experience of the learner, ultimately they know that they are not talking to a real patient. Evidence of '*conversational dominance*' may be less about the exercise of institutional power, as de la Croix and Skelton argue, and more about how participants naturally orient themselves to the particular interaction occasion.

Nevertheless, de la Croix and Skelton go on to suggest that this lack of realism should not present a major concern and typically such encounters incorporate adequate realism for the purposes of medical education. This view is, to an extent, echoed by Seale *et al.*(7), who suggest that the complexities of simulation where learners are presented with a variety of communication behaviours may in fact override the question of authenticity. Handling and negotiating these situations may encourage the development of the requisite linguistic skills for actual clinical work. Much may be learned, they argue, by the interactional work that participants undertake to sustain authenticity. Therefore, from the point of view of medical training of learner novices, the element of inauthenticity (e.g. the SP may taking a more dominant role) may actually hold some value. The idea of providing a safe environment where different communication behaviours can be explored and experimented with could actually enhance training, irrespective, they argue, of how well the simulation mimics reality.

Taking into account the arguments presented by de la Croix and Skelton and Seale *et al.*, one can, given particular circumstances, see a use for inauthenticity as a means of developing and advancing communication skills. However, in what sense can we be sure that how they interact with the learner accurately reflects typical patterns of interaction evidenced when patients attempt to take a more dominant role? Moreover, can we confidently set aside the concern over authenticity on the understanding that the SP encounter itself will encourage participants to learn and develop new communication skills which would also be helpful for the demands of medical work?

Capturing authenticity – a role for Conversation Analysis

This brings us back to the two potential barriers concerning the contextualization of learning and practice, discussed earlier. Even with the most skilful of professional actors, a simulation at best will only ever mimic authenticity. and typically how participants interact will reflect that mimicking or role-play. In thinking about maximizing authentic interaction, the problem with SP encounters, particularly when based on a real patient's story, is that the design of that role is ultimately reliant on intuitive understandings of how interaction works. However, our ordinary understandings of how talk works can often be at variance with how it actually works in context(8).

Prior to a teaching session, SPs often ask about how to raise particular topics or indeed the manner in which to raise them. These questions are important but can never really be answered satisfactorily irrespective of how familiar one may be with the particular context or indeed the particular patient's account upon which the role is based. How patients actually raise particular topics, the manner in which they raise them and how that relates to the communication behaviour of the professional are critical in identifying specific communication practices and consultation behaviours which shape these actions. Contrary to the suggestion by de la Croix and Skelton and Seale *et al.* that the pursuit of authenticity ought not to be the primary goal of the SP–learner encounter, the argument presented here proposes that authenticity of interaction is the centre point of any SP–learner encounter and that there is a real need to examine more closely the actual communication behaviours of patients when they talk to doctors to ensure a tighter integration of learning and professional aims.

Conversation Analysis is a sociological method that involves the description of the sequencing and positioning of naturally occurring talk in interactions. Application in medical encounters dates from the mid-1980s(9–11). Since then, a substantial corpus of studies has emerged, several of which concentrated on the clinical consultation. These studies have covered topics such as the overall structure of consultations(12), how patients present their problems(13), how patients convey their own explanations of the problem(14), how doctors and patients engage in question–answer sequences(11,15) and how patients respond to the way in which doctors convey a diagnosis(5,16,17). All of these studies demonstrate how the transaction of medical treatment is accomplished in and through the systematic organization of the interaction between doctor and patient.

The methodological rigour of Conversation Analysis is evident in its insistence on the empirical grounding of any description of a sequence of talk, if it is to be accepted as valid. Conversation Analysis has what might be called an in-built validation procedure where the validation or invalidation of a claim about a particular utterance can be demonstrated with reference to the next turn of talk(18). What this means is that the analyst is concerned with how interlocutors themselves display their understanding of each others' talk on a turn-by-turn basis. For example, the patient's response (verbally/non-verbally) to a doctor's diagnostic announcement displays how he/she interpreted the relevance of that announcement within the context of what is going on (Figure 7.1). This provides a useful analytical in-road to describing the systematic and organizational properties of the patient's response. More importantly, it provides something like a *'proof procedure'*(19) or validation check for any analytical claim made about the response or the overall pattern of the talk. In this way, the analysis is indifferent towards, and therefore not dependent on, the various socio-psychological dispositions of the interlocutors but is grounded in empirical observations of the talk and also shared understandings of our language practices and culture(19).

All patients are different and unique; however, once a phenomenon or practice has been identified, the analyst can then look to accumulate large collections of the same practice in order to identify its systematic properties and its regularity on particular occasions. Having established a substantial collection of examples, one can move towards a preliminary characterization of the practice in question as a first analytical step. The possibility of deviant case analysis may present itself when an example emerges that differs or indicates a departure from the identified regular practice. The *'deviant'* example can be used to underscore the systematic properties of the original identified practice and also to capture the organizational features of a variation of that practice(18), which may in turn modify the analytical claim being made.

The excerpt in Figure 7.1 comes from a study by Heath(5) who examined the interaction between doctor and patient during the diagnostic phase of the consultation. Heath observed that patients typically produced minimal responses following a diagnostic announcement from the doctor. He suggests that this phenomenon is bound up with patients' deference to clinical expertise. However, such deference, Heath argues, is also shaped by the interaction. In the excerpt below, the key communication behaviours are marked with →.

Heath notes that after the diagnostic announcement (lines 1–2), the patient declines the immediate opportunity to respond. The 1.2 second pause at line 3 (a noticeable event in ordinary talk) is designed to provide another opportunity for the patient to respond. By not responding, Heath claims, the patient displays their preference for minimal participation, restructuring the sequence of events, resulting in the doctor adding to the diagnostic announcement with a proposal for treatment and management. When the patient responds at line 6, there is another 1.2 second pause, providing another opportunity for the patient to take the floor. Again, this opportunity to contribute is declined by the patient and so the doctor continues.

Using a number of similar examples, Heath's findings draw attention to features of patients' communication behaviours and how patients use those behaviours to structure their own involvement. Heath's study shows that even when provided with an opportunity to respond, patients can withhold that opportunity, invoking interactional limits to their own participation in specific ways. Hence any interactional asymmetry or indeed *'conversational dominance'* is

Transcription symbols

° °	Talk marked by the degree sound indicates words that are softly spoken
(.)	A full stop in brackets indicates a micro pause
(1.0), (0.5)	indicates silence in seconds and tenths of seconds
[Okay	
[Yes	Talk which is preceded by a square bracket indicates overlap in speech between two different speakers

Consider the following example:

```
1.  Dr:  →   er:::::::: Yeas:: (0.3) this one's blocked
2.              (.) the other one's not.
3.        →   (1.2)
4.  Dr:      Well when would you like to have them done
5.              (.) next week some time:?
6.  P:       Yers: (.) yes please.
7.              (1.2)
8.  Dr:  →   If you'd like, to:: (.) call at um::(0.5)
9.              reception: (0.5) the girls (0.5) >on your way
10.             out (.) the girls will (0.7) sort out the
11.             appointment for you.
```

Figure 7.1 Patients' responses to diagnostic announcements.

something which is negotiated on a turn-by-turn basis. Studies such as Heath's [and more recently Robinson's(4)] provide us with a direct line of sight into actual and general communication behaviours of patients, which could be used as a basis for fine tuning SP roles and in particular patterns of communication behaviours.

Proponents of Conversation Analysis have traditionally examined naturally occurring social interaction in different social contexts since that was traditionally the primary raw data of Conversation Analysis. Part of the rationale behind this was to capture the sequential and structural rules that ordinary speakers naturally orient to in their interaction with one another. Seale *et al.*(7) used Conversation Analysis in their study and pointed out that, as a consequence of the analytical commitment to naturally occurring talk, '*artificial*' interactions in other settings (scripted speech, e.g. TV and radio) have largely remained unexamined. Yet, they argue, simulated interaction, although scripted, provides another source of interaction data that also merits investigation using this approach.

Bridging the gap between authentic and simulated interaction

How could Conversation Analysis be used to secure authenticity within the SP encounter? Stokoe(20) devised an innovative approach that utilizes the conceptual and empirical offerings of Conversation Analysis to inform role-play interaction. Stokoe's approach involves collecting audio and/or video recordings of actual interactions (e.g. between a doctor and a patient). The first step involves identifying an extract or series of extracts that demonstrate an interactional problem which may or may not lead to a successful outcome. The interaction is transcribed (using Conversation Analytic conventions). The transcript is then presented in a workshop line-by-line alongside the audio recording. After playing a short sequence, participants are asked to assess the trajectory of the interaction and provide possible solutions to the interactional problems arising.

A variety of sequences of interaction are examined in this way, providing a repertoire of actual communication behaviours. This repertoire might include how patients ask questions in a consultation, how they place and time those questions in relation to the doctor's actual communication behaviour, how patients respond to information delivery, how patients voice their information needs and participate in shared decision-making and generally how patients structure their involvement in the consultation process. The strength of Stokoe's approach is that running the audio alongside the transcript provides the context for each utterance, that is, how things are actually said. This has the added benefit of providing participants with an immediate insight into the trajectory of the interaction as it unfolds turn by turn.

For the purposes of advancing the role of the SP for medical training, Stokoe's approach could be developed further. Once a working repertoire of communication behaviours has been established from the analysis of the interaction, immersive simulation could be used to recreate key elements of the communication process of selected consultation experiences. SPs could be asked to construct scenarios based on the transcribed material and play the role of the patient based on authentic communication practices evidenced by patients in actual consultations. Calibrating each performance with the actual scenarios would

check authenticity. This process would permit a rigorous testing of various consultation scenarios to identify effective and ineffective authentic communication practices. With regard to the role of the SP, we would then be in a postion to apply those findings to demonstrate ways in which patients actually structure their involvment in the consultation process. Thus the gap between simulated and authentic interaction would be closed as a consequence of a change to SP training and role design.

This kind of approach would make significant progress in harnessing the authencity of interaction within the SP role. It would, however, be relatively labour intensive, costly and require ethical approval for the use of audio recordings of actual consultation data. At the minimum, it would require a member of staff versed in Conversation Analysis to run the data workshop. Therefore, although from an educational and professional perspective this approach to role design has much to offer, from a practical point of view it is less appealing as some of the requirements mentioned would not be easy to put in place.

A more practical alternative is probably needed that still retains the principle of using patterns of actual interaction as the guide for role design. Conversation Analysis has now built up a relatively large repertoire of studies examining how consultation behaviour is co-constructed in and through the interaction between doctor and patient. These studies (some of which are mentioned above) have generated important insights into how patients conduct themselves and interact in a variety of different clinical contexts. The many findings from this collection of research are accessible to those unfamiliar with Conversation Analysis and could also be used as a foundation for the purposes of training workshops with SPs to re-examine their role in the encounter alongside a re-examination of actual patient communication behaviours. This would be perhaps be a starting point in thinking about an applied theoretical approach for working with SPs in medical education.

Conclusion

This chapter has been designed to highlight an important but largely overlooked issue in medical education – the interactional authenticity of SP–learner encounters. Empirical findings from studies using Conversation Analysis, together with new research in this area, have been discussed as a way to harness authenticity of interaction within the SP–learner encounter. The chapter has not detailed the specifics of SP–learner encounters and how this may vary with the level of training of the novice, etc., nor has it dealt effectively with the fact that the learner enacts the role of learner within the encounter, which in itself shapes the interaction. Even real patients may take a more dominant stance when talking to a medical student than when talking to a qualified clinician. However, the use of Conversation Analysis as an approach to the role of the SP within the encounter, and the design of written SP roles, would appear to be a solid prospect in the endeavour to integrate professional and educational aims fully when SP meets learner.

References

1 Kneebone R, Nestel D, Wetzel C, Black S, Jacklin R, Aggarwal R, *et al.* (2006) The human face of simulation: patient-focused simulation training. *Academic Medicine*, **81**: 919–24.

2 de la Croix A and Skelton J (2009) The reality of role-play: interruptions and amount of talk in simulated consultations. *Medical Education*, **43**: 695–703.

3 Freidson E (1970) *Professional Dominance*. Aldine, Chicago.

4 Robinson J (2003) An interactional structure of medical activities during acute visits and its implications for patients' participation. *Health Communication*, **15**(1): 27–59.

5 Heath C (1992) The delivery and reception of diagnosis in the general-practice consultation. In: Drew P and Heritage J (eds) *Talk at Work: Interaction in Institutional Settings*, pp. 235–67. Cambridge University Press, Cambridge.

6 Murtagh GM, Furber L and Thomas AL (2013) Patient-initiated questions: how can doctors encourage them and improve the consultation process? A qualitative study. *BMJ Open*, **3** (10), e003112.

7 Seale C, Butler CC, Hutchby I, Kinnersley P and Rollnick S (2007) Negotiating frame ambiguity: a study of simulated encounters in medical education. *Communication and Medicine*, **4**(2): 177–87.

8 Schegloff EA (1996) Confirming allusions: toward an empirical account of action. *American Journal of Sociology*, **101**(1): 161–216.

9 Heath C (1981) The opening sequence in doctor–patient interaction. In: Atkinson P and Heath C (eds) *Medical Work: Realities and Routines*, pp. 71–90. Gower, Farnborough.

10 Beckman HB and Frankel RM (1984) The effect of physician behavior on the collection of data. *Annals of Internal Medicine*, **101**: 692–6.

11 West C (1984) *Routine Complications: Troubles with Talk Between Doctors and Patients*. Indiana University Press, Bloomington, IN.

12 ten Have P (1989) The consultation as a genre. In: Torode B (ed.) *Text and Talk as Social Practice*, pp. 115–35. Foris Publications, Dordrecht/Providence, RI.

13 Heritage J and Robinson J (2006) Accounting for the visit: giving reasons for seeking medical care. In: Heritage J and Maynard D (eds) *Communication in Medical Care: Interaction Between Primary Care Physicians and Patients*, pp. 48–85. Cambridge University Press, Cambridge.

14 Gill VT and Maynard D (2006) Explaining illness: Patients' proposals and physicians' responses. In: Heritage J and Maynard D (eds) *Communication in Medical Care: Interaction Between Primary Care Physicians and Patients*, pp. 115–50. Cambridge University Press, Cambridge.

15 Frankel RM (1990) Talking in interviews: a dispreference for patient initiated questions in physician-patient encounters. In: Psathas G (ed.) *Interaction Competence: Studies in Ethnomethodology and Conversational Analysis*, pp. 231–62. University Press of America, Lanham, MD.

16 Perakyla A (2006) Communicating and responding to diagnosis. In: Heritage J and Maynard D (eds) *Communication in Medical Care: Interaction Between Primary Care Physicians and Patients*, pp. 214–47. Cambridge University Press, Cambridge.

17 Maynard D (1992) On clinicians' co-implicating recipients' perspective in the delivery of diagnostic news. In: Drew P and Heritage J (eds) *Talk at Work: Interaction in Institutional Settings*, pp. 331–58. Cambridge University Press, Cambridge.

18 Perakyla A (1997) Reliability and validity in research based on tapes and transcripts. In: Silverman D (ed.) *Qualitative Research: Theory, Method and Practice*, pp. 201–20. Sage, London.

19 Pomerantz A (1990) On the validity and generalisability of conversation analytic methods: conversation analytic claims. *Communication Monographs*, **57**(3): 231–5.

20 Stokoe E (2013) The (in)authenticity of simulated talk: comparing role-played and actual interaction and the implications for communication training. *Research on Language and Social Interaction*, **46**(2): 165–85.

8 Simulated patient methodology and the discourses of health professional education

Nancy L McNaughton[1] and Brian Hodges[1,2]

[1]University of Toronto, Toronto, Canada
[2]Toronto General Hospital, Toronto, Canada

KEY MESSAGES

- Dominant ideas that underpin simulated patient (SP) methodology include competence as performance, psychometrics as a method of performance measurement and patient-centred care.
- SPs are part of a methodology that was shaped by educational needs and exist as a parallel field to medical simulation, not as one of its modalities.
- Social and cultural influences both within the health professions and in society at large have informed the development of SP methodology

OVERVIEW

In this chapter, we describe the development of SPs and their methodology over 50 years as a product of particular discourses that have dominated medical education. We use the term *discourse* as it refers to language and ways of speaking but also to 'practices that systematically form the objects of which they speak'(1). Different discourses, we suggest, have made particular practices and roles within health professional education possible for SPs. Taking a discursive approach to the subject, we identify socio-cultural influences within health professions education that have shaped the field and illustrate some of the resulting benefits and tensions for SPs and SP methodology.

Introduction

History tells us stories about events in time and the people and places attached to them often from a great height and distance, and most often as chronological accounts that point us towards eventual success (or failure). Historically, we know that the advent of SPs was the brainchild of Howard Barrows, who, in 1963, saw the effectiveness of having his neurology patients present symptoms (sometimes not their own symptoms) as a way to teach and test medical students on physical examination skills. There are many well-written descriptions of this story and of SP methodology's trajectory within health professions education(2–6).

Our intention in this chapter is slightly different and one that we hope will contribute to an appreciation for the complexity of SP methodology and the forces that have shaped it.

We are interested in the social and cultural ideas that have allowed SPs as part of a particular methodology for testing and teaching clinical skills to take hold and to thrive over the course of 50 years. The Foucauldian definition of discourse with which we are working suggests that

Simulated Patient Methodology: Theory, Evidence and Practice, First Edition. Edited by Debra Nestel and Margaret Bearman.
© 2015 John Wiley & Sons, Ltd. Published 2015 by John Wiley & Sons, Ltd.

language 'systematically form(s) the objects of which it speaks'(1). SPs, we contend, are such objects. That is to say, the notion of an 'SP' is derived from the language describing SPs and the particular practices in which they engage. Ours is a *genealogical* undertaking, which recognizes that particular practices are made possible by ways of talking, thinking and seeing. For example, different SP practices such as teaching and assessing have developed strategically in response to educational needs and changing ideas about the importance of patients as partners in their own care and the doctor–patent relationship.

In this chapter, we undertake to show how together, ideas about competency as performance, psychometrics as a measurement system and patient-centred care formed a matrix that informed the shape and possibilities for SP practice and will lead the reader through the different discourses. This is not strictly a historical undertaking in that different discourses often overlap with each other, existing co-extensively in the same place and time. However, changes in rules and practices emerge in response to social and cultural conditions, so we will be identifying the historical circumstances surrounding the different discourses and accompanying changes in SP methodology with the intention of providing a different perspective on how SPs and their methodology are situated within the larger health professional enterprise.

Competence, performance and observation

'Performance can be observed. It is about action, gesture, movement and speech and can be learned or modified through practice, repetition and the iterative loop of performance–feedback–performance'(5).

A shift within medical education in the 1960s towards a view of clinical competence as being about what one was able to *do* rather than simply about what one *knew* created a desire for new methods of teaching and testing clinical skills performance. George Miller, the main architect of this shift, argued that it was imperative that medical education move away from the assessment of knowledge ('knows') to newer methods that could assess students' actual performance of clinical skills ('shows how')(7). He created a pyramid of competencies that powerfully crystallized the idea of performance as the *central* competence. The idea that performance is essential to health professional practice created a desire for more interactive and experiential formats for learning and assessment. Live simulation as a pedagogical and assessment methodology served to support the new skills-based competencies through practice and observation and paved the way for the presence of lay persons in the medical classroom.

Performance, practice and observation were also important to Howard Barrows, the neurologist credited with the inception of live simulation and the development of the first 'programmed patient'(8). He framed his development of simulation 'as a response to the lack of observation and feedback that was endemic in medical education in the 1960s'(5). SP feedback became recognized as a valuable feature of SP simulation, coming as it did uniquely from the recipient's perspective. Like Miller, Barrows believed that observing the performance of skills was necessary for medical student appraisal and improvement. Barrows' innovation was to bring actors and models into the medical classroom. He created patient roles with accompanying symptoms, histories and physical findings that could be predetermined, providing a predictability that 'real' patients were not able to provide for a number of reasons, the least of which was their own medical conditions. According to Barrows, 'The SP … can be exactly the clinical problem the teacher wants. He can be examined serially by a number of students and present exactly the same picture and the same difficulties to every student'(8). This new technology not only allowed greater control over clinical material for teaching and testing, it also meant that students benefited from multiple observations.

The inclusion of a patient's perspective through giving feedback also created a powerful role for SPs. Feedback as a practice is based on observable behaviour and its impact on the SP. Feedback is central to the value of SPs in learning settings and to their professionalization as educators. SPs provide feedback about clinical skills, history taking, physical examination, communication and interpersonal skills(9) from the (simulated) patient's *perspective*. When providing this type of feedback, the SP focuses on how they felt during the consultation with the student and communicates constructive information about what was *observable* through both verbal and/or written mediums.

Another practice that reflected a growing patient authority was developed by Stillman, an American paediatrician. Concerned similarly by a lack of faculty observation of students' skills, she recruited and trained a group of mothers to give feedback to students on their interviews, using a process scale called the Arizona Clinical Interview Rating Scale (ACIR)(10). Stillman eventually expanded her group of teachers to include people with chronic conditions with whom she worked to develop the ability to rate not only general interviewing skills but also physical examination skills. Stillman's commitment to developing lay persons as *patient instructors* – has had far reaching effects. Patient instructors are teachers, specifically women, who provided feedback as well as acted as assessors using the ACIR scale, legitimizing their role within medical education. Not only did her early work provide a space for non-health professionals and 'real' patents in teaching and assessment, it also expanded the methodology through which SPs began professionalizing.

To summarize, the rise of a discourse of performance beginning in the mid-1960s led to specific notions about what a lay person in the medical classroom is and can be, what role they can or should play and what they are called. These names, roles and functions have propelled the legitimacy of SPs for over 50 years. The need for medical trainees to practice clinical skills as part of their developing competence and for medical educators to observe them brought performance into the classroom and contributed to new simulation practices and new subject positions for SPs.

Patient-centred discourse and communication skills

'Patient-centred care presupposes several changes in the mindset of the clinician. First, the hierarchical notion of the professional being in charge and the patient being passive does not hold here. To be patient-centred, the practitioner must be able to empower the patient, share the power in the relationship, and this means renouncing control which traditionally has been in the hands of the professional. This is the moral imperative of patient-centred practice'(11).

The emergence of the 'patient-centred' movement in the 1970s coincided with broader social changes such as increasing healthcare costs, patient consumerism, demand by patients for more egalitarian relationships with their doctors, the rise of competition from other healthcare professions, evidence-based medicine and increased surveillance of physicians by various institutions, including the government(12). Patient-centred clinical method decentres a linear objective logic with its impersonal focus on physical pathology and the doctor's implicit power, replacing it with a logic of complexity and attention to patients' suffering, emotions, beliefs and relationships. The idea of patient *care* as the main focus of clinical training rather than knowledge about disease entities has provided SPs with both an ethical and an educational rationale for their increasingly legitimate role within health professional education. This discourse, based on relationship building and a reinvigoration of the humanistic aspects of health professional practice, requires good communication skills for success and indeed for competence. Concomitant with the rise of patient-centred discourse, there has been a framing of communication as a necessary skill set, feedback as a specific developmental technique and the creation of rubrics for assessing communication skills as quality outcomes measures.

In 1991, the Toronto Consensus Conference on Doctor–Patient Communication was held, establishing a formal connection between the teaching of communication skills and clinical outcomes for patients. *The Doctor–Patient Communication: the Toronto Consensus Statement*, which came out of the conference, pulled together decades of research supporting the claims that patient complaints, missed diagnoses, patient–doctor disagreements and more are concerned 'not with clinical competency problems but with communication problems'(13).

This was part of a global health professional crisis which galvanized medical schools and licensing and accrediting organizations to focus on the public's demand for greater accountability. No longer were communication skills to be viewed as 'soft science' or were caring and compassion to be seen as peripheral to biomedical science: they would take a legitimate place beside other clinical skills needed for competent practice. These were lofty goals with interesting consequences. This rising discourse meant that it was possible to frame the value of SP work as pivotal to instilling practical skills (communication) and a general patient-centred 'know-how' in the new generation of physicians. This continues to be a key argument for the value of live simulation and SPs in medical schools, even today.

The Toronto Consensus Statement marked a threshold in medical education and had a profound impact on curriculum design, implementation, assessment and research that is still evident today. The report called for 'Highly structured programs in which specific skills are identified, demonstrated, practiced and evaluated ... ', 'development of valid and reliable assessments of communication competencies, faculty development and coherent attention ... to student's emotional issues'(13), ensuring the place and value of SPs alongside other educational essentials such as videotape, audiotape reviews and role plays as 'effective tools'.

The patient-centred discourse was also part of the rationale behind innovations such as *hybrid simulation* – mixed simulations in which a part task trainer is attached to an SP. As Bleakley *et al.* observed, ' ... colleagues promote "patient focused simulation" because they want to include authentic, context driven communication and professionalism in the learning process, bringing a human face to learning by simulation'(14).

An interesting nuance for the field of medical education is the power differential that is created by legitimizing the use of lay people for teaching in the medical academy. SPs are not, in fact, 'real' patients (with the exception of patient instructors), nor do they formally represent real patients. Indeed, it can be argued that they often portray physicians' ideas about how specific patients experience and present as 'cases'. In one of his early papers, Barrows highlighted the superiority of SPs over real patients, precisely because they *lack* individual personal characteristics(15). This is an ironic position for SPs and SP educators who have negotiated their expertise in representing and teaching about particular and different patient presentations into a place from

which to address health professional interests in 'patient-centred' care.

To summarize, a patient-centred care discourse is now deeply embedded in medicine's accountability mandate. Although the work of SPs was implicated in this emerging discourse, they did not emerge as a result of it. Rather, the rationale came afterwards. The engagement of SPs in medical schools emerged, as we have seen, to address a perception among physicians of the need for competence to be demonstrated through the performance of skills. Nevertheless, it was a short jump to extend the logic of SP methodology to align with mandates for better ways to practice, observe and measure student learning in the service of patient-centredness. Today we see similar extensions of the logic of SP-enhanced education in three newer areas of interest: inter-professional learning, patient safety and medical error disclosure. What has sometimes been more of a struggle, however, is to preserve the notion of the SP as a person rather than simply a tool or technology; a person playing a role perhaps, but one who is actively constructing a physician-patient reality.

Assessment/psychometrics

'Psychometrics is a discipline linked to psychology and statistics that is based on translating human characteristics and behaviours into numbers for comparison purposes'(5).

The discourse of psychometrics came to prominence in the 1980s. This development, together with the already operating discourses of performance and observation, resulted in a legitimizing set of assessment practices still operating within medical education today. Together, these ideas created fertile ground for new assessment technologies such as the Objective Structured Clinical Examination (OSCE), which was viewed as one of the best tools for converting student performances into numerical values. The adoption and development of OSCES in the 1970s codified the key advantages of an SP methodology identified as 'reproducible performances, easy control of content, tolerance of multiple performances and undetectability'(16). As Barrows suggested, 'One of the greatest advantages of SPs in medicine is their ability to accurately and objectively test clinical performances'(8). The observed, multistation performance examination was developed in order to measure student performance, determine the effectiveness of teaching methods and provide the basis for a fair, objective, reliable, repeatable and valid appraisal of student performance(17). Many terms have been used in the literature for multiple station performance-based examinations, but the OSCE has won out as the most recognizable name for this technology. No longer a novelty at the end of the second decade of the twenty-first century, OSCEs have been widely implemented by health professions around the world and remains one of the more researched and reported on technologies in medical education.

During the last two decades of the twentieth century, the influence of medical educators with training in psychometrics led to a much greater emphasis on standardization, reliability and validity in assessment. With the rise of psychometrics, new venues and processes were necessitated for assessing student performance and also new roles for clinical faculty and SPs observing and measuring these performances. *SPs* were transformed into *standardized patients*. As Wallace noted in her 'History of standardized patients in medical education', the term *standardized* became generally accepted when the focus of medical education research 'turned sharply toward research clinical performance evaluation'(3).

Psychometrics and assessment not only changed the activities in which SPs took part but also provided a platform from which this group of educators could further professionalize within health professions education. With increasing demand for performance assessments across a range of health professions and to assess a number of different skill sets, SPs currently perform as assessment *instruments* for observing faculty, but have, in some places, become the assessors of clinical skills in their own right. The latter development had led to a proliferation of training and evaluation processes to ensure their *accuracy*. In the 1970s, Harden and colleagues in the United Kingdom could scarcely have imagined that the OSCE would become a tool for national licensing and an entrance to practice for foreign trained clinicians, but this is exactly what happened when it was taken up by large testing organizations and further developed to serve psychometric purposes. Today, OSCEs have been rigorously modified to create maximal standardization and reliability. The regimented rotation, the strictly standardized test measures and the collection of massive amounts of data have become a testament to the dominance of the psychometric discourse to the extent that these OSCEs bear only a passing resemblance to the first examination Harden created for medical students(5).

At a socio-cultural level, the local, regional and national differences between OSCEs are relevant to an examination of SP methodology. Most evident are the different roles made possible within the OSCE *cultures* that have become strikingly different from one country to another. There are specific ideas about who should be authorized to act as an assessor in OSCEs that can be examined through a cultural filter. For example, economic priorities of efficiency and cost savings mean that in the United States, standardized patients are framed as being more readily available and less expensive than physician examiners. Thus SP examiners are the foundation of the whole United States Medical Licensing Examination system (Clinical Skills Assessment). By contrast, in Canada and the United Kingdom, there has been an effort to maintain the role of the physician examiner in OSCEs. This framing rests on arguments about *professional judgement* of competence by peers, a tradition of *volunteerism* in medical education and less priority given to psychometrics than to *authenticity*(18).

To summarize, an assemblage of technologies was put in place with the introduction of OSCEs, including standardized patient role creation, techniques for role training, standardizing roles, enacting roles and creating assessment tools such as checklists and observation protocols, all of which placed SPs at the centre and increasingly as leaders in simulation as an educational assessment methodology. SP involvement in assessment has been a main component for a distinct *standardized* branch of SP methodology, creating new, powerful roles for SP educators within health professions education. SP educators are working in leadership positions in large national health professional licensing organizations such as the American National Board of Medical Examiners, the Medical Council of Canada and the Education Commission on Foreign Medical Graduates, and are among the decanal leaders of medical schools. Psychometric discourse and the standardized assessment branch of the SP family have unquestionably brought opportunities; they have also created some tensions with SP engagement as creative artistry in the services of learning.

Conclusion

SP methodology has developed over 50 years in response to social and cultural influences that were supportive of a newly legitimizing field of medical education. The ways in which the methodology has been taken up and the practices made possible for SPs have varied across time and location. This is explained to some extent by the dominance of different discourses, including competence as performance, of psychometrics and of patient-centred care. Here we have tried to illustrate how these different discourses create opportunities but also tensions.

Roles for SPs continue to change along with the evolution of the field of healthcare education, creating new opportunities for SPs as educators, administrators, consultants and scholars.

Further developments in the field of SP education, such as hybrid and immersive large-scale and disaster training simulations, are indications of a methodology that is still successfully adapting to varying educational and professional training needs so many years after its inception. As is discussed by others in this book, SP-based education has now expanded to include professional development and education for fields beyond health professional practice.

As a closing note, we would like to underscore the extent to which thinking about SPs as a *tool* or a technology 50 years after their creation is insufficient. SP educators and in many cases SPs themselves have a wealth of expertise that encompasses both clinical and lay knowledge about what constitutes competent practice, including of course the components and organization of clinical interviews, physical examination techniques and the affective elements of a medical interaction. Today, SP educators also act as facilitators of simulation learning, sometimes alongside clinician teachers and sometimes alone. They work with both students and practising professionals. They work with medical students and physicians but also with all of the other health professionals and many other professional groups as well. SP educators design curricula and create initiatives and innovations using their knowledge of SP practice as both a technology and as a methodology. The shift from being thought of as a tool for *'teaching about'*, to being engaged as educators who have control of their own technology and methodology in order to *'teach with'* is an important professionalizing moment. Today, SPs and SP practices do not represent another modality within the broader simulation field: they contribute through their rich and well-developed educational methodology to the advancement of health professions education.

References

1 Foucault M (1980) *Power/Knowledge Selected Interviews and Other Writings 1972–1977.* Random House, New York.
2 Barrows HS (1987) *Simulated (Standardized Patients) and Other Human Simulations.* Health Sciences Consortium, Chapel Hill, NC.
3 Wallace P (1997) Following the threads of an innovation: the history of standardized patients in medical education. *Caduceus*, 3(13): 5–28.
4 Adamo G (2003) Simulated and standardized patients in OSCEs: achievements and challenges. *Medical Teacher*, 25(3): 262–70.
5 Hodges BD (2009) *The Objective Structured Clinical Examination: A Socio-History.* Lambert Academic Press, Cologne.
6 May W, Park JH and Lee JP (2009) A ten year review of the literature on the use of standardized patients in teaching and learning: 1996–2005. *Medical Teacher*, **31**: 487–92.
7 Miller G (1990) The assessment of clinical skills/competence/performance. *Academic Medicine*, **65**(9): S63–7.
8 Barrows HS (1971) *Simulated Patients (Programmed Patients): Development and Use of a New Technique in Medical Education.* Thomas: Springfield, IL.
9 Stillman PL, Regan MD, Philbin M and Haley HL (1990) Results of a survey on the use of standardised patients to teach and evaluate clinical skills. *Academic Medicine*, **65**(5): 288–92.
10 Stillman P, Brown D, Redfied D and Sabers D (1977) Construct validation of the Arizona clinical interview rating scale. *Educational and Psychological Measurement*, **7**: 1031–8.
11 Stewart M, Brown JB and Freeman T (2003) *Patient-Centred Medicine: Transforming the Clinical Method.* Radcliffe Medical Press, Abingdon.

12 Castellani B (2006) The complexities of medical professionalism. In: Wear, D. and Aultman J (eds) *Professionalism in Medicine: Critical Perspectives*, pp. 3–23. Springer, New York.

13 Simpson M, Buckman R, Stewart M, McGuire P, Lipkin M, Novack D, *et al.* (1991) Doctor–Patient Communication: the Toronto Consensus Statement. *BMJ*, **303**(6814), 1385–97.

14 Bleakley A, Bligh J and Browne J (2011) *Medical Education for the Future: Identity, Power and Location*. Springer, Dordrecht.

15 Barrows H (1993) An overview of the uses of standardized patients for teaching and Evaluating Clinical Skills. *Academic Medicine*, **68**(6): 443–51.

16 Sanson-Fischer RW and Poole RD (1980) Simulated patients and the assessment of medical students' interpersonal skills. *Medical Education*, **14**(4): 249–53.

17 Harden RM and Gleeson FA (1979) Assessment of clinical competence using an observed structured clinical examination. *Medical Education*, **13**(4): 1–47.

18 Hodges B and McNaughton N (2009) Who should be an OSCE examiner? *Academic Psychiatry*, **33**: 282–4.

Part 3
Educational Practice

9 Preparation: developing scenarios and training for role portrayal

Debra Nestel[1], Carol Fleishman[2] and Margaret Bearman[1]
[1]Monash University, Clayton, Australia
[2]Johns Hopkins Medicine, Baltimore, USA

KEY MESSAGES

- Cases or scenarios provide the clinical and educational contexts for simulated patient (SP)-based simulations.
- Real patients can make a significant and direct contribution to scenario development.

- Templates provide valuable guidance in developing scenarios and SP roles.
- A four-stage model – person, learning activity, context, rehearsal – provides a systematic and person-centred approach to training SPs for role portrayal.

OVERVIEW

This chapter outlines two important elements for working within SP methodology. Both are associated principally with the preparation phase – developing scenarios and training SPs for role portrayal. Underpinning the chapter is the notion that SPs are proxies for real patients and, as such, finding ways to connect *real* with *simulated* patients is part of SP methodology. We argue that those who write SP roles (ourselves included) are often distanced, as a consequence of our professionalization from the experiences of real patients. Real patients can contribute to scenario development. We propose a four-stage model to training SPs for role portrayal. This approach centralizes the *person* (patient) during the training ensuring that the character of the person to be portrayed remains prominent, allowing the group of SPs to develop a shared and coherent understanding of the SP role, the scenario and the overall activity.

Introduction

This chapter addresses two important elements for working within SP methodology: scenario development and training for role portrayal. Both of these belong primarily in the *preparation* phase (Figure 1.1). Like many aspects of simulation, different terms are used to describe practices. We use the terms *scenarios* and *cases* interchangeably to describe the educational and clinical contexts, which form the simulation encounter. We distinguish the *SP role* of portraying a specific patient from the scenario. For example, the patient

Ms Shannon Betts may have many encounters with health and social care services. Each one of these encounters can become a scenario. Ms Betts might go to a general practice clinic and be assessed by a nurse practitioner (communication and physical examination scenario); she may require an intramuscular injection (professionalism and procedural skills scenario in hybrid simulation); or be seen by a physiotherapy student learning about postoperative care (clinical skills scenario). An advantage to thinking about SP roles in this way is that it focuses on the patient rather than the clinical skill. The processes that we

Simulated Patient Methodology: Theory, Evidence and Practice, First Edition. Edited by Debra Nestel and Margaret Bearman.
© 2015 John Wiley & Sons, Ltd. Published 2015 by John Wiley & Sons, Ltd.

describe support this patient-focused approach(1) to simulation-based education.

Approaches to scenario development

Writing the scenario or SP role

It is valuable to think about scenario and SP role development as a multistage process. The driver for the scenario usually comes first and may be an assessment requirement, a gap in provision of care, patient safety concerns or as part of an overall curriculum. There is surprisingly little published literature on processes for writing scenarios. The nature and purpose of the scenario will always determine the details. However, based on experience, the following practices are useful: be systematic by using a template; consider multiple perspectives – patients, learners, clinicians or specialists; keep the language and format of the scenario simple so that it is appropriate for SPs rather than healthcare professionals; and focus on key information, keeping the role within a couple of pages. When thinking about scenario development, it is worth mentally rehearsing what is expected to happen in the scenario and to check these expectations against resources (e.g. funding, rooms, personnel, props, time). Do this early on, as scenarios must be feasible.

Planned scenarios are most commonly used in SP-based education, although *improvised* scenarios are also possible. Even though authors are generally SP educators or clinicians, other educators such as specialist faculty (e.g. communications, ethics, patient safety, counsellors) may also contribute. Team of authors are common, particularly with respect to interprofessional scenarios. Direct involvement of patients, families or advocates is likely to result in truly patient-centred SP roles and more authentic representation of the patient's point of view.

Real patient perspectives

SP roles and scenarios are usually based on real patient experiences as *interpreted* by clinicians or SP educators. A scenario may derive from several patients' experiences forming a composite role or be completely fictional. SP educators and clinicians, by virtue of becoming a member of their profession, no longer experience healthcare as *ordinary* patients. The personal accounts of clinicians who become patients attest to the different lenses through which the service is experienced(2–4). Without real patient involvement, SP-based work is 'a mirror for the teachers' preconceptions rather than as an authentic reflection of a patient encounter'(5). Snow (Chapter 14), an *expert* patient who has observed simulation educators at work, noted, '…the patient voice continues to be filtered through clinicians' perspectives'.

Chapters 14 and 15 provide excellent illustrations of ways in which real patients can author or contribute to scenario development. Likewise, Nestel *et al.* invited volunteer SPs (unpaid and with no prior experience with this work) to write their own roles(6,7). The learning objective was to provide novice medical students with an opportunity to practice and reflect on their ability to use basic interviewing skills in a clinical context. The volunteers were asked to think about a recent encounter in family medicine and then populate a scenario template. These volunteer SPs then portrayed themselves in this simulated scenario with the medical students. The SP educators found the scenarios to be fascinating due to the variations inherent in the lived experiences of the volunteers. Some of the SP roles have also been re-used as is, whereas others were modified, for different scenarios.

Another approach is to interview real patients with the disclosed intent of crafting scenarios based on their experiences. Capturing each patient's verbal description of their ideas, concerns, need for information and expectations addresses patient-centeredness directly(5,8,9). There are a small number of studies in the literature illustrating the value of this approach(10,11). In one such study, Nestel and Kneebone noted that many SP roles were single problem and did not reflect the experiences of patients with complex histories(5). Patients known to faculty were selected and invited to participate in interview sessions at the medical school, where the patients were individually asked to tell their story of their illnesses to the SP educators. Information from this interview was used to populate a template with the purpose of creating scenarios to teach senior medical students how to conduct patient-centred interviews and consider the clinical management of patients with complex histories. The real patients were invited to review the scenarios and to attend the training sessions.

The whole process proved salutary, especially for the SPs who were directly connecting with those for whom they were proxies. The SPs were able to ask questions of the patients regarding their illnesses and thus were able to better understand their situations.

Involving real patients may be impractical to do for all scenarios, but it is a valuable process and goes some way to ensuring that SPs are proxies for real patients and not simply agents of the SP educator or clinician. In the above example, care was taken to address ethical concerns and volunteers and patients were fully informed of the faculty's intentions. Identities of patients, clinicians and sometimes institutions were changed to maintain confidentiality.

Documenting and reviewing scenarios and SP roles

Scenarios may be documented in many forms. They are usually textual but may also include audiovisual illustrations. Documentation establishes enduring shareable resources that represent significant investments and achievements. The documentation process allows the developers to 'articulate' and critically reflect on their simulation practice. The process also facilitates quality assurance such as mapping simulations against curriculum goals.

Commonly, documentation involves using some kind of template. SPs usually need access to both the scenario and the SP role and they are usually incorporated into one document. Templates contain an outline of the typical elements of a scenario. The benefits of using templates for scenarios include: recording and presenting information in a structured and systematic way; easy comparison of scenarios; cross-referencing to curriculum and clinical practice standards or competencies; promoting reflection on simulation practice; and supporting new simulation educators in developing their practice. The limitations of using templates include: restricting creativity and flexibility. There is no single template available for all simulation modalities, although there are common elements (Box 9.1). For SP roles within the scenario, there are additional elements (Box 9.2).

Scenarios and SP roles should also be reviewed during the *evaluation* phase for areas in which to make improvements such as meeting the learning

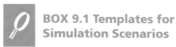

BOX 9.1 Templates for Simulation Scenarios

Scenario development details

- Name of scenario (patient name and may include their illness or the relevant clinical skill)
- Author(s) of scenario
- Date of development
- Process for development

Brief summary/overview
Scenario purpose

- Intended learner group (description)
- Overall aim
- Learning objectives
- Context of the simulation (formative or summative assessment, etc.)

Logistics

- Number of participants
- Type of participants
- Equipment required
- Consumables required
- Safety/risk (to participants and others)
- Length of simulation
- Number and arrangement of chairs/tables/exam tables

Briefing

- Instructions to all participants including learner's tasks

Simulation activity

- Starting state
- Finishing cue
- Time out option and signal

Debriefing and assessment

- Feedback/debriefing approach
- Assessment instruments

Reflection

Evaluation

BOX 9.2 Additional Elements for the SP Role in Scenario-Based Simulations*

1. Summary/overview including patient's characteristics (name, age, sex, appearance)
2. Setting
3. Patient's affect/behaviours
4. Opening lines/questions/prompts
5. Patient's reason for interaction (presenting problem), including their ideas about the problem, their concerns and expectations
6. Patient's history of the problem
7. Patient's past medical history
8. Patient's family medical history
9. Patient's social information (work, lifestyle, habits)
10. Considerations in playing this role including wardrobe, makeup, challenges

*Roles are powerful when they are written in the second person. For example: 'Your name is Louise MacIntosh. You have come to the general practice because you have been getting headaches. You work part-time in your local supermarket and really enjoy it because many of the staff have worked there for a long time too and have become your friends'.

objectives and fitting the timing available. A review framework, drawn from a conceptual framework of writing effective cases(12), is provided in Box 9.3.

BOX 9.3 Review Framework for Simulation Scenarios

Structural Elements

- Review *relevance*
  - What are the learning outcomes, learner level, and and scenario setting?
  - Who are the SP and the learner portraying and what is the emotional intensity of the encounter?
  - Do the structural elements align?
- Review *authenticity*
  - What sources informed the scenario development and how does the SP role reflect the experiences of real patients?
  - What sources informed the scenario development and how does the SP role reflect the experiences of real patients?
  - What complexities/nuances are present and do they match the level of the learner?
  - What 'gaps' in realism are the learners required to overcome and are they reasonable?

Process Elements

- Review *engagement*:
  - How will the learner know what to do or say at the start or at any given point in the scenario?
  - How do learners' actions change the SPs' responses and/or the outcome of the scenario?
  - How do learners interact with each other?
- Review the *level of challenge*:
  - What skills or tasks do learners have to do that they have not already done? How will you account for this?
  - How will learners know the requirements of the scenario?
  - How do you know that the learners will have sufficient 'headspace' to learn from the scenario (e.g. will not be overwhelmed by a challenging SP role)?
  - How will SPs adjust as needed, to different levels of competency?

Outcome Elements

- Review *educational* design
  - How is the learner's performance assessed? What is the SP's role in this?
  - How does the scenario link with briefing, debriefing and reflection phases?
  - How and when does feedback occur? What is the SP's role in this?
  - How does the scenario link in with prior knowledge and/or overall curriculum?

Source: Adapted from the NHET-Sim Program materials(15).

Crafting SP roles on the run

In some sessions, SP roles, and sometimes scenarios, are crafted with faculty and learners to meet specific requirements of the learners. This approach draws on the experiences of learners and usually requires experienced SPs. This enables the educational experience to be tailored to the needs of the participants and often draws on the learner's experiences. The amount of *improvisation* required during performance relates to the way in which the SP role or scenario is constructed and more rapid, less focused SP training may be required.

Training for role portrayal

There are many approaches to training SPs for role portrayal and surprisingly few with an evidence base. We describe a four-stage model, which draws from the dramatic arts theories(13,14) in addition to practical experience. The four stages are illustrated in Figure 9.1 and involve (1) development of the person's character, (2) explaining the learning activity to the SPs, (3) exploring the clinical context and (4) rehearsing.

In the following, each phase is outlined. The person leading the training is referred to as the SP practitioner. It is optimal to have SPs seated in a horseshoe with a white board (or flip chart) as a central focus and to explain the process to them prior to commencing. It is assumed that SPs will have had an opportunity to read the role. Box 9.4 provides an overview of the process.

1. **Person phase** This phase places the first and intrinsic value on the *person*, that is, the patient to be portrayed, without reference to their illness or purpose in the scenario. In this phase, the SPs do most of the talking. SPs are asked to consider two questions that define the essence of the person to be portrayed (Box 9.4). Alternatively, the practitioner can ask the SPs to *free associate*, by calling out words that come to them when they think of the person to be portrayed in a state of wellness. All responses are recorded on a white board. This shared visual field is a valuable aide memoire as the training progresses, enabling SPs to put aside the written role. Once the free association starts to slow down, the practitioner asks the SPs to identify any responses that they disagree with or are ambivalent about. This permits early

identification of different interpretations of the role; these differences can be discussed with a view to developing a shared understanding. This may be by SP negotiation or, in the case of high-stakes assessment, it may be directed by the SP practitioner.

2. **Learning activity phase** During the *learning activity* phase, the SP practitioner does most of the talking. The practitioner outlines the details of the scenario. The following topics could be addressed: characteristics of the learner group, such as professional discipline or level of experience; the purpose of the learning activity including learning objectives: nature of the learning activity and whether it is formative or summative assessment; logistics such as time or repetitions; feedback requirements; and the role of faculty. It can also be helpful to demonstrate briefly the simulation encounter, possibly by video or audio recording, to let the SPs know the endpoint of training.

   Depending on the learning activity and the experience of the SPs, this phase takes up to 10 minutes. It is important not to make assumptions that the SPs will know about the learning activity or understand their role within it. If SPs work across several programmes and/or participate in many different types of simulation activities, it is easy for them to forget the nuances that can influence the success of a learning activity. The information is critical to successful portrayal.

3. **Context phase** During the *context* phase, the SPs move to thinking about the person as a patient. The SP practitioner asks questions that articulate the facts of the scenario (Box 9.4) and returns to the white board to record the SPs' responses. This phase ensures that the SPs have a sense of the patient's perspective about their health issue. The white board serves as a summary. Using visual methods, such as concept mapping, can be helpful and 're-presenting' the data in this way can reinforce content. This process usually takes about 10 minutes but depends on the complexity of the scenario and the experience level of the SPs. The context phase provides an opportunity for clarification and/or negotiation of content.

4. **Rehearsal phase** The *rehearsal* phase serves to integrate the previous three phases and contains four processes. In the first round, all

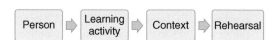

Figure 9.1 Phases for training SPs for role portrayal.

BOX 9.4 Aims, Topics and Examples of Questions Addressed in each Phase for Training SPs

Phase 1: Person
Aim: To develop a shared understanding of the identifying characteristics of the person to be portrayed as a patient

- The SP practitioner asks:
  - Who is the person separate from their illness?
  - How would you describe their personality?

Phase 2: Learning activity
Aim: To develop a shared understanding of the purpose and logistics of the simulation activity

- The SP practitioner describes the simulation as a learning or assessment activity and then seeks questions from SPs to ensure the purpose and logistics are understood.

Phase 3: Context
Aim: To develop a shared understanding of the *person* in a clinical context

- The SP practitioner asks:
  - Why is this person in this clinical scenario?
  - What facts are important in this clinical scenario?
  - What is the patient's understanding of their healthcare issue?
  - What are the patient's main concerns?
  - What is the patient's most likely outcome in this context?
  - What is this patient's current emotion? Why? How will it be presented?
  - What is the most likely patient behaviour throughout the scenario?
  - What clinician behaviour will influence the patient's emotion? How?

- May include a demonstration, orientation to setting, etc.

Phase 4: Rehearsal
Aim: To practice the role to ensure portrayal is within the expected *bandwidth* for the person

- In the first round, the SP practitioner asks:
  - Where do you live? Alone? How long have you been there?
  - Can you tell me about your family? Your parents? Your siblings?
  - Where do you work? Do you like it? What do you like about it?
  - Can you describe a typical day at work?
  - How would you describe your diet?

- In the second round, the SP practitioners ask about clinical information while the SP takes on the emotional affect of the patient:
  - Why have you come to the health service today?
  - Can you give me some more information?
  - What do you think is causing your health problem?
  - What are you concerned about?
  - What are you expecting will happen?

- In the third round, the SPs do a partial rehearsal with a competent learner using a rotating hot seat method (20–30 seconds each SP) increasing to 45–75 seconds as portrayal is calibrated.

- In the fourth round, learners with varying skills interact to enable the parameters of portrayal to be observed, demonstrated and practiced.

SPs assume the role of the person simultaneously. The SP practitioner asks questions about the person, while the SPs all respond in role. The SP practitioner moves from one SP to the next maintaining a tempo to keep all engaged.

The questions (Box 9.4) help the SPs assume a shared interpretation of the person they are portraying. In the second round, the SP practitioner asks SPs to assume the initial emotional state of the patient at the commencement of the scenario. The goal is to calibrate expression across SPs so they perform similarly. The SP practitioner then asks questions about relevant clinical information in a similar manner to the first round. In the third round, the setting for the scenario is approximated and the opening minutes of the scenario are enacted, with one SP playing a competent learner and another starting off in the 'hot seat', that is, playing the role of the SP. After the scenario has played out for a short period, the SP practitioner calls 'swap'. The next SP takes the patient 'hot seat' and aims to continue in the scenario as if nothing has changed, until the next 'swap' is called. Initially these swaps are done every 20–30 seconds, and then after some discussion and calibration by SPs and the SP practitioner (about 2 minutes into the encounter) the time periods for each SP are lengthened to 45–75 seconds. If the opening is performed as intended, then the rest of the scenario is likely to flow well from the SPs' perspective. This approach requires SPs to pay attention to all facets of the portrayal. To test the parameters of the SPs portrayal, this can be repeated with *learners* of various skills and attitudes.

The fourth and final round consists of further practice, with SP observers providing feedback to each other. Once the performance is consistent and the SPs have no further questions, then the SPs are ready for the simulation.

Benefits and challenges of the four-stage model
The first and foremost benefit to this four-stage model is that the person is at the centre of the training. This reflects patient centredness and allows the same SP role to be trained for multiple scenarios, in a range of professional contexts. This is an important economy. Second, the systematic approach provides SPs and SP practitioners with a structure for a complex process and provides a shared, coherent understanding of the SP role and scenario. Finally, SPs who become used to working with the model can become SP practitioners, allowing for SP-led training.

Challenges in using the model occur when the scenario or role is poorly developed or that information is not available to SPs prior to training. Additionally, the model is optimal for use with a group size of six and it can be time consuming.

Training for role portrayal on the run
As mentioned earlier in the chapter, there are circumstances when roles are created at the time of the learning activity. This may be to re-enact an encounter which a learner would like to rehearse managing better. Box 9.4 serves as a guide to the type of information that the SP would require; the SP would usually work with the learner(s) and SP practitioner directly to discuss this information. There may be partial rehearsal to ensure the SP's portrayal is appropriate and then the rest of the interaction is improvised. This approach can be challenging for inexperienced SPs and those who are not professional actors.

Giving feedback on role portrayal
In many respects, training for role portrayal is a continuous process since SPs value and benefit from feedback on their portrayal to make improvements. This means that faculty or SP practitioners need to observe and provide feedback during/after the learning activity. This would usually take place in the *debriefing/reflection/evaluation* phases (Figure 1.1).

Conclusion
In this chapter, we have focused on two elements of working within SP methodology – scenario development and training for role portrayal. We highlighted the role of the patient voice in both processes. In scenario development, patients can be valuable contributors to creating roles and are likely to have an authenticity that clinician-crafted roles do not. In training, the SP role is independent of the scenario and training methods allow the person and person's experience to be highlighted rather than the clinical concern. Finally, it is worth noting that each programme, SP practitioner and group of SPs is unique and the appropriate variations on these methods and other methods are encouraged.

References
1 Kneebone R, Nestel D, Wetzel C, Black S, Jacklin R, Aggarwal R, *et al.* (2006) The human face of simulation: patient-focused simulation training. *Academic Medicine*, **81**(10): 919–24.
2 Jones P (2005) *Doctors as Patients*. Radcliffe Publishing, Abingdon.
3 O'Brien C (2008) *Never Say Die*. HarperCollinsPublishing, Sydney.

4 Klitzman R (2007) *When Doctors Become Patients*. Oxford University Press, New York.

5 Nestel D and Kneebone R (2010) Authentic patient perspectives in simulations for procedural and surgical skills. *Academic Medicine*, **85**(5): 889–93.

6 Nestel D, Tierney T and Kubacki A (2008) Creating authentic simulated patient roles: working with volunteers. *Medical Education*, **42**(11): 1122.

7 Nestel D, Tierney T, Muir E and Kubacki A (2008) Learning to talk with patients: feasibility of a volunteer simulated patient programme for first year medical students. *International Journal of Clinical Skills*, **2**(2): 121–8.

8 Nestel D, Cecchini M, Calandrini M, Chang L, Dutta R, Tierney T, *et al.* (2008) Real patient involvement in role development evaluating patient focused resources for clinical procedural skills. *Medical Teacher*, **30**: 795–801.

9 Nestel D and Bentley L (2011) The role of patients in surgical education. In: Fry H and Kneebone R (eds) *Surgical Education: Theorising an Emerging Domain*. Springer, Dordrecht.

10 Black SA, Nestel DF, Horrocks EJ, Harrison RH, Jones N, Wetzel CM, *et al.* (2006) Evaluation of a framework for case development and simulated patient training for complex procedures. *Simulation in Healthcare*, **1**(2): 66–71.

11 Kneebone R and Nestel D (2010) Learning and teaching clinical procedures. In: Dornan SE, Mann KV, Scherpbier JJA and Spencer JA (eds) *Medical Education: Theory and Practice*, pp.193–210. Churchill Livingstone Elsevier, Amsterdam.

12 Kim S, Phillips W, Pinsky L, Brock D, Phillips K and Keary J (2006) A conceptual framework for developing teaching cases: a review and synthesis of the literature across disciplines. *Medical Education*, **40**(9): 867–76.

13 Stanislavski C (1936) *An Actor Prepares*. Routledge, New York.

14 Spolin V (1999) *Improvisation for the Theater*, 3rd edn. Northwestern University Press , Evanston, IL.

15 Bearman M and Nestel D (2014) *Module S10: Developing Scenarios*. Health Workforce Australia, Melbourne.

10 Simulated patients as teachers: the role of feedback

Debra Nestel[1], Margaret Bearman[1] and Carol Fleishman[2]
[1]Monash University, Clayton, Australia
[2]Johns Hopkins Medicine, Baltimore, USA

 KEY MESSAGES

- Feedback can be conceptualized as a dialogue, which supports self-regulated learning.
- Simulated patients (SPs) offer feedback from patient perspectives.
- SPs need to be supported in feedback practices.

- SPs can be educated to offer feedback with respect to patient centredness and communication.
- Debriefing is generally faculty led, draws from a number of models and is strengthened by including SPs.

OVERVIEW

This chapter presents the case for SPs providing feedback from their unique perspective within the simulation encounter. Feedback is generally considered key to learning in simulation and SPs can be supported to develop their feedback skills, particularly in the areas of patient-centred care and communication. We blend the use of theory, empirical evidence and practice guidelines. We offer approaches to facilitation that are inclusive of SPs.

Introduction

SPs are often thought of synonymously with 'role portrayal', but this focus on performance overlooks significant additional contributions. One of the SP's most important roles is to teach through feedback. In this educative role, the SP is an expert who can deepen the learner's understanding of the patient's experience. This unique perspective is one of the great advantages of SP methodology over alternative simulators.

SPs often, although not always, provide feedback through a faculty-led debriefing process. This chapter commences with an overview of various aspects of SPs' feedback, with particular emphasis on the ways in which SPs can support learners in improving their patient-centred care. This feedback is then explored within the context of broader debriefing practices.

SPs and feedback

In the education and simulation literature, one of the most important elements of facilitating learning is described as feedback(1). Historically, feedback has been considered to be the transmission of information from one person (usually an expert) to another (usually the learner). However, in higher education, feedback is increasingly thought of as a two-way process(2), and the overlap between conceptions of feedback and debriefing is similarly growing. The role of the SP in debriefing is discussed later in this chapter.

Feedback is sometimes referred to as *closing the loop* in learning or exposing the gap between the actual and expected performance(3). For SPs, it may be helpful to think of feedback as identifying the gaps between what they expected in the encounter and what they experienced.

Simulated Patient Methodology: Theory, Evidence and Practice, First Edition. Edited by Debra Nestel and Margaret Bearman.
© 2015 John Wiley & Sons, Ltd. Published 2015 by John Wiley & Sons, Ltd.

Another way of thinking about feedback is that it should support and develop the learners' capacity to regulate their own learning(3). Nicol and Macfarlane-Dick(4) outlined seven principles of good feedback which support self-regulation and we consider these with respect to SP-based education (Table 10.1).

In SP-based education, the facilitator and SP may offer feedback verbally, via rating forms, or by a combination of each. All of these modes involve the SP making complex judgements about the learner's performance. Even though feedback can be through verbal or written commentary, one form of written feedback, rating forms, provides more limited information about possible improvements since it precludes dialogue. Here our focus is on feedback which promotes learning, rather than summative rating.

One of the benefits of working with SPs is that they are able to provide feedback on patient centredness. Stewart referred to patient-centred care as when the clinician has achieved 'an integrated understanding of the patient's world', that is, the whole person including their emotional needs and life issues(5). Patient-centred clinicians seek common ground with the patient on their *problem* and mutual agreement on management, prevention and health promotion. It has been noted with some irony that patient centredness, when explicitly taught, is usually explained by those most likely to be distant to its experience – clinicians(6). Observing encounters from the outside, from the clinician/faculty

perspective, can look and feel very different to the SP and learner experience within the encounter. When SPs provide feedback, they do so as proxies for patients and are therefore in a strong position to offer feedback that clinicians may be less able to provide(7–9).

There is some debate about whether the SP stays 'in role' for feedback. Staying in role (that is, in character) has many limitations, especially if the patient being portrayed is arrogant or non-communicative, thus impeding learning. We recommend that the SP clearly steps out of role by introducing themselves to the learners. The SP can then share their experience of the learner from their unique viewpoint, which is both 'inside' and 'outside' of the encounter.

Training SPs to offer feedback

Feedback is described as 'hard to give and hard to take'(6), and learning how to give feedback on patient centredness is not necessarily intuitive but is complex and requires specific skills. SPs should be supported in gaining these skills through training. First, SPs should become familiar with principles of patient-centred care and effective communication skills. Encouraging SPs to think about answers to the following questions can help them think about targeted feedback for patient-centred communication. The questions are adapted from those designed for clinicians reflecting on their patient centredness(10):

Table 10.1 Application feedback principles(4) in SP-based education.

Feedback principle	Application in SP-based education
1. Clarify what good performance is	Ensure the SP and the learner know the expected level of performance (e.g. patient-centred communication skills).
2. Facilitate self-assessment	The facilitator and the SP can ask the learner questions to promote reflection and probe reasons for their behaviour (e.g. When you were asking me why I came to see you, you only followed up on the first thing I said. I wonder why you did this?)
3. Deliver high-quality feedback information	The facilitator and SP need to provide feedback that relates to predefined criteria; is timely; includes information on strengths/weaknesses and corrective advice; prioritizes areas for improvement; and is available for learners to access for future reference
4. Encourage facilitator and peer dialogue	The facilitator should enable SPs and learners to discuss their respective experiences
5. Encourage positive motivation and self-esteem	Facilitators and SPs should leave learners inspired to improve their practice and maintain existing positive qualities
6. Provide opportunities to close the gap	Facilitators can provide an opportunity for the learner to immediately rehearse with the SP the proposed communication strategies – even in a partial format. Facilitators can discuss ways in which the learner might practice the learning point elsewhere
7. Use feedback to improve teaching	Facilitators and SPs can reflect on their own practices in facilitation, in offering feedback and for the SP in role portrayal

- How did I feel throughout the encounter?
- What did the learner do that led to my satisfaction?
- What did the learner do that led to my feeling dissatisfied?
- Did I feel listened to?
- Did I get the chance to share my ideas?
- Was I able to share my concerns?
- Was I given a chance to ask questions?
- Did I feel comfortable enough to ask questions?

- Was I given the opportunity to make specific requests?
- Were my feelings acknowledged?
- Did I feel respected?
- Was I treated as an individual?
- Did I seem important or valued?

Giving SPs a list of communication skills can provide them with the language to describe to learners the impact of specific communications on them during encounters (Box 10.1). Once SPs have

---

 BOX 10.1 Examples of Communication Skills SPs may Describe in Offering Feedback to Learners

Commencing the encounter

Greet the patient
State your full name
Clarify your role
Obtain the patient's name
Attend to the patient's comfort
Obtain the patient's consent
State the purpose of the interaction
Mention note taking
Clarify the time available
Assess the patient's ability to communicate
Demonstrate interest and respect
Empower the patient to ask questions or seek
    clarification of anything that is unclear

Gathering information

Use open questions initially
Allow the patient to complete first sentence(s)
Identify the patient's ideas, concerns and
    expectations
Use active listening – verbal (e.g. staying with
    patient's topic; using patient's words; reflection)
    and, non-verbal (e.g. eye contact; nodding)
Use other non-verbal behaviours (e.g. body posture;
    gestures; facial expressions, nodding)
Use open-ended questions and move towards
    closed ones as appropriate
Pick up verbal and non-verbal cues
Probe sensitively
Survey for other problems
Signpost or transition statements
Set an agenda
Make interim summaries

Giving information during the encounter

Establish baseline knowledge
Relate information to patient's ideas, concerns and
    expectations
Give specific rather than general advice
Use emphasis to highlight key points
Use repetition to highlight important information
Chunk information into usable bits of information
Check patient understanding

Closing the encounter

Provide an end summary
Discuss an action plan
Check for further information
Ask for questions
Check if the patient has any worries or concerns

Relationship-building skills

*Throughout each stage, it is important to use
    relationship-building skills in order to establish and
    maintain the relationship with the patient*
Use active listening
Make empathic statements
Show warmth
Pick up verbal and non-verbal cues
Use non-verbal behaviours (e.g. posture, gestures,
    facial expressions)
Identify the patient's ideas, concerns and
    expectations

*Not all the skills listed here will be used in every interaction
The skills are not necessarily in a specific order, although
some skills obviously precede others*
    Adapted from program materials developed by the
first author with colleagues at Imperial College
London

been familiarized with concepts of patient centredness and relevant communication skills, they are well equipped to develop their feedback skills.

There are a number of different approaches to training SPs in developing their feedback practices. A valuable method is to work with a group of SPs and to watch a recording of an SP-based encounter together as the basis for several exercises. These might include the following:

- *Using a rating form*
  After orientating the SPs to a rating form, ask the SPs to imagine they were the SP in the encounter and complete the form. Encourage them to use the whole scale. Facilitate a group discussion to help SPs identify the similarities and differences in their judgements.
- *Writing feedback*
  It can be helpful to ask SPs to write the words they would use when giving feedback. These phrases can then be collated as 'sound bites' for other SPs. It helps to expand the vocabulary and precision of SP feedback. However, it is important that the SP feels comfortable with 'owning' them.
- *Completing the sentence*
  Valuable feedback from the SP includes expression of emotions in response to learner actions. Support the SPs in achieving this through activities such as asking the SP to complete the following sentence, 'I felt (*INSERT FEELING*) when you said/did (*STATE WORDS/ACTIONS*)'. Make a list of the *feeling* words the SPs might use and do this exercise routinely.
- *Feedback monologue*
  Another useful activity following a group viewing of an SP-based encounter is to ask the SP to rehearse condensed verbal feedback. Ask the SPs to imagine they are the SP in the video and that they will be asked to give feedback to the learner. Brief the SPs on the scenario, including the learning objectives and the characteristics of the learner. Encourage the SPs to take some notes while they are watching (even though they cannot do this in real practice). After viewing the video, ask the SPs to think for a few minutes about the feedback they would provide to the learner. Working in pairs, ask one SP to give feedback to their partner (who role plays as the learner although they are not permitted to speak). The verbal feedback should be completed in 90 seconds. After this

first round, discuss the content and how the experience felt for the SP and the *learner*. In the second round, swap roles, incorporating ideas from the small group discussion. The drill is helpful in structuring content, practicing precision in language and observing the impact on learners, although it is different from the usual practice in that it is a monologue. The process can also serve to calibrate SPs' feedback. Box 10.2 provides two examples.

Table 10.2 sets out some of the challenges associated with SPs offering feedback. Most of the challenges are addressed through thoughtful and regular training opportunities for SPs and, where possible, offering joint facilitator and SP training.

The debriefing framework

Debriefing is considered a vital component of simulation (see Figure 1.1); it is the mainstay of team-based simulations and is also widely practised in SP-based education. SPs often, but not always, provide feedback within a debriefing framework. Debriefing usually takes place immediately after a simulation and it may comprise a small group facilitator-led discussion involving the SP and the learner(s) from the simulation and may include other learners (as observers in the simulation). There are many models or approaches to debriefing, which are well described in the healthcare simulation literature(11–17). In most of these approaches. the facilitator can offer the SP an opportunity to give specific feedback, in addition to the SP participating in most of the other discussion activities that take place during the debriefing. It is helpful to think of the SP as a full member of faculty and to include SPs in planning, implementing and evaluating debriefing sessions. Box 10.3 offers a detailed structure for an SP-based debriefing and draws on a Pendleton approach(18).

The Calgary–Cambridge Observation Guide is an approach to debriefing developed for patient-centred communication encounters. It is commonly applied in SP-based encounters with the SP joining the debriefing as a full participant. The key steps in facilitation are as follows:

1. Start with the learner's agenda.
2. Always look at the outcome you are trying to achieve.

BOX 10.2 Two Examples of SP Feedback in this Drill

Example 1: Monologue after SP-based encounter on patient-centred interviewing

'Louise, I really enjoyed our encounter even though my character and the scenario were quite challenging. The key thing was I felt listened to because you stayed with the topics I raised, especially in the beginning of the encounter. You asked me thoughtful questions that clarified my sometimes jumbled story telling and that also helped to make me feel valued and respected. Your tone of voice, your pace of speech, few interruptions and that you stayed silent for a few seconds when I was in story-telling mode made me feel important. I felt really comfortable to ask questions, too, and so I was able to ask you about whether I really should be worried about my headaches. That was a key concern for me. I wonder if you could think of better ways to deal with my concern – perhaps telling me that it was at least a good step I had taken to visit the doctor so we could investigate, rather than offering me what might turn out to be false reassurance. Think about why you said everything would be alright – I have the impression it made you feel better rather than really attending to me. You demonstrated some really fine skills and I hope you can take some time to think about the conditions that led to you using them and think of the reasons why you offered what might be false reassurance so you can avoid that in future.'

Example 2: Monologue after SP-based encounter on hybrid simulation for procedural skills

'Thanks for that. I am sorry I don't know your name. I don't think you introduced yourself. I'd like to give you some feedback from my perspective. I thought you did well overall. The things that you did that were helpful for me are: First, using my name at the beginning of the scenario and then again at the end – it felt like I was an individual – it really personalized the experience. Second, asking me what I already knew about the procedure – I think it meant we were more efficient together. Third, shaking my hand when you left – again, it just felt personal. Parts of our interaction where I felt less connected to you were, first, I think I missed some important information when you were speaking quickly at the beginning of the consultation. I was trying to get used to your speaking voice and your fast pace of speech made this hard for me. Second, when you were having trouble getting your gloves on you let your frustration show – I was losing confidence in you – I was thinking that if you couldn't get your gloves on, I didn't really want you sticking needles into me. Saying something like, "The gloves stick when your hands are wet" and smile or something like that would be reassuring. And finally, you seemed to just run out of the room when you finished. That was odd since you had given me so much time at the beginning (even though you spoke really quickly), I was anticipating a little more time with you but you were off. I hope you take some time to think about these points. It might be helpful to think about how you were feeling in the consultation when you did the things I have described. Thanks.'

3. Encourage learner self-assessment and problem solving.
4. When working in groups, get everyone involved in problem solving.
5. Provide balanced feedback.
6. Make offers and suggestions.
7. Rehearse suggestions.
8. Be well intentioned, valuing and supportive(19).

One approach used in immersive simulations is called *pause and discuss*. In these simulations, the scenario is *paused* either by the learner or the facilitator and a brief discussion ensues that addresses a key learning point. Learners are made aware of the process during briefing. Discussions can include explaining decisions, use of techniques, considering next steps and so on. Although SPs do not usually initiate a *pause*, they may be asked to contribute to the discussion.

BOX 10.3 Framework for Debriefing an SP-Based Session on Patient-Centred Interviewing

Session involves one facilitator, one SP and four learners

Briefing

- Welcome learners
  - Identify the first learner to conduct the patient-centred interview
  - Discuss the learning objectives including specification of the expected performance
  - Conduct a 10 minute patient-centred interview with an SP
  - The interview will be recorded and clips used during the debrief
  - Immediately after the interview, the learner returns to the debriefing room where they will be asked how they felt during the interview, what they thought went well and what could be improved
  - The SP's experience of the interview will be shared in relation to the expected performance
  - Observers are asked to note specific elements of performance for sharing in the debriefing
  - The facilitator will also offer feedback
  - A summary will be made of the learning (nominate one or two observer students to do this)
- Brief the learner on the SP and their specific task
- Ask the learner if they have any questions
- Ask if there are any particular skills they would like observed
- Offer to knock on the door at eight minutes to indicate two minutes remaining
- Ensure recording equipment is switched on

Simulation activity

- Learner conducts the interview
- Facilitator and other learners observe the encounter
- Note particular time frames to review

Debriefing

- Immediately after the encounter, when the learner and the SP return to the debriefing room, follow the sequence below and be flexible in attending to the learner's needs

- Facilitator asks the learner:
  - Can you very briefly state how you felt during the encounter?
  - Can you name two skills that you used that worked well? Why?
- Facilitators asks the SP:
  - Can you identify two skills that the student used that were effective? Why?
- Facilitator asks the observers if they would like to add to these skills
- Facilitator can add to these skills
- Facilitator asks the learner:
  - Can you name two skills that you would like to improve?
- Facilitator asks the SP:
  - Can you identify two skills that the learner could have used to improve the encounter? Why?
- Facilitator asks the observers if they would like to add to these skills
  - Designated learner shares ratings from rating form
- Facilitator can add to these skills
- Review 2–3 short clips of the encounter
  - Involve the learner, SP and observers in a discussion of the clips
- Involve the group in making recommendations for improvements
- Rehearse one of the recommendations, if desirable
- Summarize the debriefing
- Ask the learner if they have any further questions
- Repeat the process for all learners building on each interview

Reflection

- Learners complete a written reflection after the session and to plan *how* and *when* they will check if they have achieved the learning objectives

Evaluation

- SP and learners complete a written evaluation form on the value of the session

Table 10.2 Challenges and strategies associated with SPs offering feedback.

Challenge	Strategies
The SP is not invited to give feedback	Provide facilitators with opportunities to observe SP feedback so they can learn how work with and value SPs during the debriefing
The learners are not prepared for feedback from SPs	Brief learners thoroughly as to what the SPs will be doing and their role in providing feedback
The SP is not prepared to give feedback	Offer training to SPs on feedback and ensure they are fully briefed about what they will be expected to do and assist them during exercises with preparing their feedback
The learner has done a really good job and the SP does not think there is much to say	Explain to the SPs that it is still important to offer information on what has been done well so the learner keeps their skills
The learner has performed poorly and there is a lot to give feedback on	Explain to the SPs that it is important not to give too much information – they should identify about three priorities and just focus on those items
The learner leaves feeling flat and/or uninspired	Review the feedback with the SP and encourage them to reflect on the words they used and give the SP feedback on their feedback
The SP leaves feeling flat and/or uninspired	Debrief the SPs to explore what transpired during the simulation practice
The facilitator and learner did not value the feedback	Ensure that facilitators and learners are oriented to the role of SPs and provide SPs regular training to ensure they offer meaningful feedback
It is difficult to find appropriate feedback phrasing to address areas for the learner to improve	Carry out drills and exercises with the SPs
The SP gives feedback from a clinician's perspective instead of from a patient perspective	Provide opportunities for SPs to reflect on their feedback by regularly reviewing of their practice and considering if it is from the patient's perspective

Another approach is called *Plus Delta*. The facilitator conducts a *brainstorming* activity immediately after the simulation in which learners' reactions are quickly recorded on a shared visual field (e.g. white board, flip chart). These are divided into *Plus* – things that have worked well, and *Delta* – things that could be improved or be changed. The group generates as many ideas as possible and then selects a few to focus on exploring in detail. Selection usually aligns with the intended learning objectives. The approach is valuable when time is short and SPs can participate during the brainstorming and the deeper exploration.

Video-assisted debriefing

Video-assisted debriefing (VAD) refers to the use of video in debriefing. Although there is evidence for some VAD practices associated with simulation, it is usually in the context of manikin-based simulations. The increasing ease of image capture and review of videos is likely to lead to more use in SP-based simulations. However, ensuring VAD has a positive impact on learning requires careful consideration. Thought needs to be given to camera and microphone placement. SPs need to be briefed on seating arrangements to capture their

BOX 10.4 Benefits of Video Recording in SP-Based Simulations

- Documenting the encounter for immediate or later review
- Enabling learners to see themselves as others might see them
- Showing learners what they have done well to reinforce effective performance
- Showing learners what they might improve (e.g. speaking too quietly, closed postures)
- Assisting recall of learners, SPs and faculty
- Prompting discussion
- Considering time related elements of the encounter
- Assuring quality SP performance

facial expressions, body positioning and verbal exchanges with learners. Some of the benefits of recording SP-based simulations are summarized in Box 10.4.

It is helpful for facilitators and SPs to take a few moments immediately after the simulation to identify specific clips to review. The clipsare often used as a trigger for discussion. It is helpful when the facilitator or SP *frames* the clip by letting the learners know what they are about to see and what they should look for when they are watching. Using just two or three short clips, of 30–45 seconds each, in a debriefing session is usually sufficient. In some programs, learners are provided with their own recording for later review and as evidence for portfolios. There are also administrative considerations such as permission for the use of images. Participants and SPs should be informed of the intention to record, why and what will happen with the recording after the simulation, and in some instances written consent may be required.

Conclusion

Feedback is often identified as the single most important element that supports learning in a simulation. SPs have an important and unique contribution in offering feedback to learners. SPs act as proxies for real patients, allowing learners to hear about the patient's experiences and feelings from *inside* the encounter. SPs can be supported through training to develop feedback skills on patient centredness and relevant communication skills. Feedback and debriefing can be conceptualized as a multidirectional flow of information and SPs can support the development of self-regulatory behaviours in the learner. Debriefing is usually faculty led and is most effective when it includes the SP.

References

1 McGaghie WC, Issenberg SB, Petrusa ER and Scalese RJ (2010) A critical review of simulation-based medical education research: 2003–2009. Medical Education, **44**(1): 50–63.
2 Molloy E and Boud D (2013) Changing conceptions of feedback. In: Boud D and Molloy E (eds) *Feedback in Higher and Professional Education: Understanding It and Doing It Well*, pp. 11–33. Routledge, London.
3 van de Ridder JM, Stokking KM, McGaghie WC and ten Cate OT (2008) What is feedback in clinical education? *Medical Education*, **42**(2): 189–97.
4 Nicol D and MacFarlane-Dick D (2006) Formative assessment and self-regulated learning: a model and seven principles of good feedback practice. *Studies in Higher Education*, **31**(2): 199–218.
5 Stewart M (2001) Towards a global definition of patient centred care. *BMJ*, **322**(7284): 444–5.
6 Bleakley A and Bligh J (2008) Students learning from patients: let's get real in medical education. *Advances in Health Sciences Education*, **13**(1): 89–107.
7 Kneebone R, Nestel D, Wetzel C, Black S, Jacklin R, Aggarwal R, *et al.* (2006) The human face of simulation: patient-focused simulation training. *Academic Medicine*, **81**(10): 919–24.
8 Nestel D and Bentley L (2011) The role of patients in surgical education. In: Fry H and Kneebone R (eds) *Surgical Education: Theorising an Emerging Domain*, pp. 151–68. Springer, Dordrecht.
9 Nestel D and Kneebone R (2010) Authentic patient perspectives in simulations for procedural and surgical skills. *Academic Medicine*, **85**(5): 889–93.
10 Robertson K (2014) *Communication Skills*. BMJ Learning, http://learning.bmj.com/learning/module-intro/communication-skills-guide.html?moduleId=6057021 (accessed 15 April 2014).
11 Rudolph JW, Simon R, Dufresne RL and Raemer DB (2006) There's no such thing as 'nonjudgmental' debriefing: a theory and method for debriefing with good judgment. *Simulation in Healthcare*, **1**(1): 49–55.
12 Rudolph JW, Simon R, Rivard P, Dufresne RL and Raemer DB (2007) Debriefing with good judgment: combining rigorous feedback with genuine inquiry. *Anesthesiology Clinics*, **5**(2): 361–76.
13 Raemer D, Anderson M, Cheng A, Fanning R, Nadkarni V and Savoldelli G (2011) Research regarding debriefing as part of the learning process. *Simulation in Healthcare*, **6**(7): S52–7.
14 Jeffries PR and Rogers KJ (2007) Theoretical framework for simulation design. In: Jeffries PR (ed.) *Simulations in Nursing Education: from Conceptualization to Evaluation*, pp. 21–58. National League for Nursing, New York.
15 Dreifuerst K (2010) Debriefing for meaningful learning: fostering development of clinical reasoning through simulation. PhD thesis, Indiana University Scholar Works Repository.
16 Imperial College London (2012) *The London Handbook for Debriefing: Enhancing Performance Debriefing in Clinical and Simulated Settings*. Imperial College London, London.
17 Howley LD and Martindale J (2004) The efficacy of standardized patient feedback in clinical teaching: a mixed methods analysis. *Medical Education Online*, http://med-ed-online.net/index.php/meo/article/view/4356 (accessed 5 July 2014).
18 Pendleton D, Schofield T, Tate P and Havelock P (1998) *The Consultation: an Approach to Learning and Teaching*. Oxford University Press, New York.
19 Silverman J, Kurtz S and Draper J (2005) *Skills for Communicating with Patients*, 2nd edn. Radcliffe Publishing, Abingdon.

11 Teaching and learning physical examination skills with simulated patients

Anna K Vnuk

Flinders University, Adelaide, Australia

 KEY MESSAGES

- Physical examination (PE) is a complex process that can be learned in several ways – with real patients, peers, manikins and task trainers and simulated patients (SPs).
- SPs can make a significant contribution to teaching PE skills.
- SPs supporting learners in the development of PE require careful screening and training.
- Ensure processes are established for referring SPs who have unexpected clinical findings.
- SP-specific scenarios that reflect their personal PE findings offer valuable learning experiences.

OVERVIEW

Physical examination (PE) is a complex and essential component of work in many health professions. Patients, when conscious, have an important role to play in this examination process. However, real patients are often compromised in this role owing to their state of wellbeing. This chapter explores contemporary approaches to teaching health professional students about PE, including learning with real patients in clinical settings, with peers in a skills laboratory, with manikins and task trainers and with SPs in simulated clinical settings. The recruitment, screening and training of SPs are outlined. Ways of supporting SPs in offering feedback to learners on PE are described. Developing SP-specific scenarios that reflect their PE findings can offer learners a rich and authentic experience.

Introduction

This chapter describes how SPs contribute to the development of physical examination (PE) skills in learners. PE is a complex psychomotor task, used to assess the wellbeing of patients and to assist with clinical decision-making, in relation to the diagnosis. Information from history taking can lead to a diagnosis in up to 80% of patient presentations(1,2). PE is therefore used to confirm or refute diagnoses. The health professional learner must decide what signs would be present in a patient with each of the possible diagnoses and so determine which body systems to examine, which region to concentrate on and whether any special examination tests or manoeuvres must be undertaken(3). Before starting, the learner must explain the purpose of the examination to the patient and obtain consent. Additionally, each part of the examination should be at least briefly explained and specific instructions offered on how to breathe, which way to move and more(4). The patient should be continuously monitored by the learner for any signs of discomfort and the examination altered or negotiated according to the patient's

Simulated Patient Methodology: Theory, Evidence and Practice, First Edition. Edited by Debra Nestel and Margaret Bearman.
© 2015 John Wiley & Sons, Ltd. Published 2015 by John Wiley & Sons, Ltd.

responses. The examination should be performed in a technically correct fashion, in order to elicit signs which must be identified, characterized and interpreted by the learner, in the light of the possible diagnoses(5). On the basis of these findings, further examination may be added. Investigations may be required to confirm the diagnosis(1,2). The examination findings and likely diagnoses are explained to the patient (and reported to the examiner in an assessment or teaching situation). On the basis of the likely diagnosis, management options should be discussed and negotiated with the patient. It can be seen that PE consists of a complex list of tasks: cognitive, physical and communicative, balancing the need to obtain information for the diagnosis with patient comfort.

Current methods of teaching PE

There are two major steps involved in teaching PE – demonstration and practice – and these can occur in different ways.

1. **Real patients in clinical settings:** The advantages of this method are considerable(6) as this is authentic learning. As the patient is presenting with a real problem to be resolved, the opportunity exists for learners to experience PE findings which are congruent with the presenting condition and so to develop a personal memory(7,8) of the characteristics of the PE signs: how an enlarged liver feels, what swollen ankles look like, what a pleural friction rub sounds like. However, there are significant disadvantages with teaching on real patients at the bedside. There are well-documented difficulties in finding patients who are willing and able to withstand PE by multiple learners(9). Examining a patient at the bedside also leads to a significant disruption to the doctor–patient interaction by the addition of multiple learners whose needs are considerable and often in conflict with those of the patient. Monrouxe *et al.*(10) suggested that the patient is often relegated to the status of a 'prop', that is, the patient is usually not involved in the interaction between the learners and the doctor and is only 'used' to demonstrate signs which are then discussed, often with medical jargon, leaving the patient open to potential confusion and concern about their condition.

Additionally, the patient may be exposed for long periods of time(10). Being treated as a 'prop', being talked over and being exposed are all demonstrations of poor role modelling of patient-centred care by the doctor. Examination of patients by learners who are inexperienced may lead to increased discomfort by patients. However, patients do volunteer for PE and one of the reasons expressed is to find out more about their medical condition by listening to the discussion about their condition between the doctor and the learner(11).

2. **Peers in the clinical skills laboratory setting:** This is a time-efficient and cost-effective method for practising PE as learners are always present and are not paid to be models for each other. Peer PE is claimed to promote empathy(12) and to provide a safe learning environment for learners(13). Additionally, in a multicentred study(14), there was almost universal acceptance by learners of examining and being examined by other learners in at least one body region. However, there are also some disadvantages. During peer PE, the learner being examined has no health problems that need resolving, making the situation *artificial*. Even though learners may have abnormal PE findings(15), these are uncommon and there is an expectation that there will not be abnormal findings. This can affect the learners' understanding of the purpose of PE, which is, of course, to look for diagnostic evidence, leading instead to the learners *going through the motions* of PE and not engaging in the task(16). Also, during demonstration to the group by the tutor and during group practice in peer PE, students may feel compelled to participate and/or to disrobe more than they would prefer, particularly male students for examinations involving the front of the chest(16). Cultural barriers may also preclude peer PE. Further, when learners examine each other, the examinee can anticipate the instructions(16), which actually prevents the examiner from developing their skills in clear communication of instructions and explanations.

3. **Manikins and task trainers:** The use of manikins and task trainers in learning PE is generally limited to providing learners with experiences of abnormal PE findings, for example, heart sounds and murmurs. The advantage of not causing harm to patients

is compelling, but equally, manikins do not encourage learners to develop interpersonal skills with the patient. Additionally, some task trainers do not represent valid findings(17) and so may not assist the learners in developing accurate skills and perceptual and interpretative abilities.

Teaching and learning PE with SPs

SPs address many of the difficulties generated by teaching and learning with real patients, peers, manikins and task trainers. SPs prevent harm to patients and can provide a safe learning environment for learners and patients. SPs also allow fair examination privileges for learners of both genders and all cultures. Although SPs do not provide authentic learning, the artificial situation can be used to advantage. This includes stopping and starting of the PE to correct errors, questioning and probing to check and deepen understanding. The development of realistic scenarios can expand knowledge and skills, particularly in clinical reasoning. SPs can participate in demonstration, rehearsal and assessment.

Recruitment of SPs

Potential SPs need to be properly briefed and screened before training and work.

1. SPs need to have the teaching or assessment activity clearly explained to them, particularly what will be required of them in terms of undress, physical contact and any intrusive *poking*. For example, feeling for sacral oedema requires the learners to expose the base of the spine, an area usually covered by underwear. SPs also need to know the length of hours of work and likely number of learners, so that they can make a decision about their perceived physical endurance for the task.

2. Each SP needs to have a medical history and an examination performed on them by a member of staff who is a practising doctor with medical indemnity insurance. This also permits the potential SP to make an informed decision about what they are willing to have examined and if there are any limits that they wish to impose. For example, some female SPs do not like to be used for heart and lung examination because of the potential for too much palpation around the breast. If any unknown medical condition or sign is uncovered, SPs are referred

to their GP for follow-up. Although it is not the role of clinical academic staff to treat the SPs, they still have a duty of care to ensure that any condition or abnormality uncovered by clinician examination or learner examination is followed up. To this end, in our department, a form is kept and the SP is asked at a later date if they have followed up the referral, but not what the outcome is, as this is confidential. Additionally, knowing about the PE findings of the SPs allows decisions to be made about which teaching and assessment situations they would be most suited for. Some SPs (like real patients) have PE signs that are harder to elicit than others, so, for example, we prefer not to include SPs with very quiet heart sounds in assessments for early learners.

3. SPs are reminded that the PE performed by learners does not count as *proper* PE. For example, if they have been asked to return to their GP for a check-up, they must still maintain at arrangements with their doctor.

Once an SP has accepted an offer of employment, they need training for their role.

1. At the simplest level of training, we ask the SPs to respond to learners' questions as if they have never had the examination done before and so they should take the instructions literally. For example, if the learner asks the patient to hold their breath, they will continue to do so until they are told to breathe again. If the instructions are unclear or too quiet, the SP should not guess or anticipate but ask for them to be repeated clearly.

2. In response to inappropriate behaviour by learners (e.g. rudeness), the SP should look surprised or offended and, if necessary, make comment on this within their role. For example, if learners forget their introductions, the SP should ask them who they are.

3. At the end of the examination, the SP can give generic feedback about the PE to either the learner or the tutor about the clarity of instructions or roughness and discomfort (e.g. 'Your finger nails were digging into me').

This training is important because otherwise the SP may have a tendency to become the *professional patient* who anticipates the learners' instructions. This would put the SP–learner interaction at the same level as peer PE, which might prevent the learner from developing communication skills.

In a typical teaching activity, a tutor and SP demonstrate the examination with the advantage that the tutor can take their time demonstrating, knowing that the patient is robust enough to endure the examination for this length of time and can cope with multiple examinations from learners. However, good role modelling should still be maintained by the tutor, checking on patient comfort and covering the patient up to prevent cold, discomfort and embarrassment. The SP can also support learners in practising their PE skills, particularly under the supervision of the tutor. Time can be taken to give feedback to the learners to help refine their skills and to get feedback from the patient on any discomfort produced. The learners can be questioned to help integrate the skills with the underlying knowledge, without concerns about worrying the patient by use of confusing jargon. However, this is also a great opportunity to teach learners about terms that can be used in front of the patient and how to explain to the patient using lay terms. These sessions are also an opportunity to get feedback on the communication from the SP in role as patient. Box 11.1 sets out a generic plan for involving SPs in a PE teaching session.

BOX 11.1 Example of a Teaching Session for Medical Students Learning PE

- Overall aim: To teach and assess PE.
- Learning objectives

  Primary

  - Demonstrate the technical skills required for successful PE.
  - Demonstrate communication and patient interaction skills (including instructions and explanations of findings).
  - Raise awareness of patient's perspective during PE (particularly with regard to discomfort).

  Secondary

  - Describe and practise diagnostic decision-making and clinical reasoning (development).

- Target participants: Medical and other health professional learners, particularly those learning PE in the preclinical years of their course. When a tutor demonstrates PE with an SP, the approach

works effectively with up to eight students around the bedside. An SP with advanced training could work alone with up to four students.

- Setting: Clinical skills laboratory settings (presence of a bed and curtain for privacy).
- Programme/Session length: 1–3 hours.
- Faculty (number and experience): One clinical tutor for each SP, unless the SP has been trained to teach and give feedback on PE teaching and assessment, then the ratio can be decreased, with one tutor present to clarify any questions about PE which are outside the areas that the SPs have been trained in and to generally supervise the teaching by a number of SPs.
- Simulator(s): Simulated patients.
- Frequency of offering: Variable. Some tutors may wish to have SPs present for every session of PE, particularly if the decision has been made not to use peer PE. Others may include SPs just for demonstration of a new skill and/or for assessments.

The SP can also participate in assessment of PE. The advantage is that the same patient can be a *standardized* assessment for learners, without a real patient being *over examined* or potentially abused.

The role of the SP can be developed to *value add* to both the teaching and assessment of PE:

1. **Increasing the level of feedback to the learners** Over time, and with training and feedback, the SP can develop skills so that they can give feedback to the learner on the technical aspects of the skill, particularly those palpation skills that can be assessed from the patient's perspective (e.g. 'your hands are in the wrong position to feel the kidney', or 'you didn't press deeply enough during deep palpation'). This requires training, feedback from, and discussion with, the tutor. This feedback can be a very useful adjunct to the tutor's own feedback. With further training, SPs can develop the skills to be able to assess and give feedback on PE[18] without the need for the tutor to be observing every SP–learner encounter. We ask SPs to give detailed feedback on a checklist for each encounter and, with training and feedback on standard setting, they are comfortable in making a global rating on the performance. We use video to capture the encounters and review

the videos of those students that the SPs rate as 'fail' or 'unsure'. We also view a selection from all SPs as a quality control. This saves faculty time (and money) while ensuring that all learners are competent in basic PE skills(19).

2. **Adding history taking to the PE** If history taking is added to the PE, this can develop and assess clinical reasoning skills. However, active questioning of the learners about their thought processes is required, as clinical reasoning is more frequently assessed through discussion(20), so that, after the history taking, the learner should be asked what they think the likely diagnosis could be and what they expect to find on PE, or this can occur after the SP encounter, during review of the video(21).

If we wish the learners to engage fully in looking for the PE findings that are likely to be present on a patient with their history (which is what happens in clinical practice), then it becomes important that their PE findings be congruent with the history. For example, if the patient gives a history of the development of right heart failure but then on examination has no peripheral oedema or raised jugular venous pressure, then it does not teach the learners to engage in looking for signs on the PE and they begin to ignore obvious findings or assume everything will be normal(22). This may lead to learners developing bad habits in PE or not understanding the role that PE plays in assisting with the process of coming to a likely diagnosis. This is where it is possible to develop authenticity by incorporating the SP's PE findings (uncovered in the pre-employment PE) into the patient's scenario – with the patient's permission, of course. For example, an SP who had gastro-oesophageal surgery (a Nissen fundoplication) many years ago had a scenario created for him of a *patient* who had reflux surgery that was unsuccessful and had lived with reflux for years but was now presenting with increasing dysphagia, and the learners need to consider diagnoses such as stricture or oesophageal carcinoma. This encourages the learners to take into account all of the PE findings (in this case, the presence of a large central upper abdominal scar) because they are all congruent with the patient's history. Another example is to use the presence of mild pitting oedema on an SP to create the scenario of a patent with mild right heart failure. For SPs with minimal abnormal PE signs (including younger SPs), scenarios can be created of patients with paroxysmal conditions (e.g. asthma, palpitations) or they can be trained to simulate abdominal pain. This prevents the PE from being a performance and encourages the learners to integrate their skills and knowledge. In effect, these assessments become like 'long cases'(23), but the difference is that a real patient is not required, the content and level of difficulty can be standardized between learners and the learner–patient interaction is observed.

Conclusion

SPs can make an important contribution to teaching and learning about PE. Their involvement in teaching and assessment prevents harm to real patients, while enabling the SPs to give learners an insight into patients' perspectives. It also provides a fair learning experience for all learners. The role of the SP can be developed to provide feedback on the technical aspects of the task to the learners and also to assess learners, leading to cost savings. Scenarios can be developed that increase authenticity and permit the development and testing of clinical reasoning skills, rather than just a focus on technical performance of PE skills. However, local guidelines must be developed to prevent negative health outcomes for the SPs (and the potential litigation of clinical academics), and include screening of all SPs, referral to a health provider to follow up any problems uncovered and reminders about the continuation of routine health checks.

References

1 Hampton JR, Harrison MJ, Mitchell JR, Prichard JS and Seymour C (1975) Relative contributions of history-taking, physical examination and laboratory investigation to diagnosis and management of medical outpatients. *BMJ*, **2**(5969): 486–9.

2 Peterson MC, Holbrook JH, Von Hales D, Smith NL and Staker LV (1992) Contributions of the history, physical examination and laboratory investigation in making medical diagnoses. *Western Journal of Medicine*, **156**(2): 163–5.

3 Benbassat J, Baumal R, Heyman SN and Brezis M (2005) Viewpoint: suggestions for a shift in teaching clinical skills to medical students: the reflective clinical examination. *Academic Medicine*, **80**(12): 1121–6.

4 Silverman J, Kurtz S and Draper J (2005) *Skills for Communicating with Patients*, 2nd edn. Radcliffe Publishing, Abingdon.

5 Sibbald M, Panisko D and Cavalcanti R (2011) Role of clinical context in residents' physical examination diagnostic accuracy. *Medical Education*, **45**: 415–21.

6 Nair BR, Coughlan JL and Hensley MJ (1997) Student and patient perspectives on bedside teaching. *Medical Education*, **31**: 341–6.

7 Duvivier R, Stalmeijer RE, van Dalen J, Van der Vleuten CPM and Scherpbier AJJA (2012) Influence of the hospital workplace on learning clinical skills. In: Duvivier R (ed) *Teaching and Learning Clinical Skills. Mastering the Art of Medicine*, Uitgeverij BOXPress: s-Hertogenbosch.

8 Cox K (1998) How well do you demonstrate physical signs? *Medical Teacher*, **20**: 6–9.

9 Olson L, Hill S and Newby D (2005) Barriers to student access to patients in a group of teaching hospitals. *Medical Jounal of Australia*, **183**(9): 461–3.

10 Monrouxe L, Rees C and Bradley P (2009) The construction of patients' involvement in hospital bedside teaching encounters. *Qualitative Health Research*, **19**: 918–30.

11 Chretien KC, Goldman EF, Craven KE and Faselis CJ (2010) A qualitative study of the meaning of physical examination teaching for patients. *Journal of General Internal Medicine*, **25**(8): 786–91.

12 Braunack-Mayer A (2001) Should medical learners act as surrogate patients for each other? *Medical Education*, **35**: 681–6.

13 Wearn A and Bhoopatkar H (2006) Evaluation of consent for peer physical examination: students reflect on their clinical skills learning experience. *Medical Education*, **40**(10): 957–64.

14 Rees CE, Wearn AM, Vnuk AK and Sato TJ (2009) Medical students' attitudes towards peer physical examination: findings from an international cross-sectional and longitudinal study. *Advances in Health Sciences Education: Theory and Practice*, **14**(1): 103–21.

15 Pols J, Boendermaker P and Muntinghe H (2003) Incidence of and sequels to medical problems discovered in medical learners during study related activities. *Medical Education*, **37**: 889–94.

16 Vnuk AK (2013) Going through the motions: medical students' experiences of learning physical examination (unpublished doctoral dissertation).

17 Macintosh M and Chard T (1997) Pelvic manikins as learning aids. *Medical Education*, **31**: 194–6.

18 Stillman PL, Regan MB, Swanson DB, Case S, McCahan J, Feinblatt J, *et al.* (1990) An assessment of the clinical skills of fourth-year students at four New England medical schools. *Academic Medicine*, **65**(5): 320–6.

19 Hasle JL, Anderson DS and Szerlip HM (1994) Analysis of the costs and benefits of using standardized patients to help teach physical diagnosis. *Academic Medicine*, **69**(7): 567–70.

20 Pulito AR, Donnelly MB, Plymale M and Mentzer RM Jr, (2006) What do faculty observe of medical students' clinical performance? *Teaching and Learning in Medicine*, **18**(2): 99–104.

21 Rose M and Wilkerson L (2001) Widening the lens on standardized patient assessment: what the encounter can reveal about the development of clinical competence. *Academic Medicine*, **76**(8): 856–9.

22 Hauer KE, Teherani A, Kerr KM, O'Sullivan PS and Irby DM (2007) Student performance problems in medical school clinical skills assessments. *Academic Medicine*, **82**(10 Suppl): S69–72.

23 Norcini JJ (2002) The death of the long case? *BMJ*, **324**(7334): 408–9.

12 Simulated patient methodology and assessment

Cathy M Smith[1], Carol C O'Byrne[2] and Debra Nestel[3]

[1]University of Toronto, Toronto, Canada
[2]Pharmacy Examining Board of Canada, Toronto, Canada
[3]Monash University, Clayton, Australia

 KEY MESSAGES

- Simulated patients (SPs) are the 'examination question' in performance assessments and therefore need to be 'standardized' in order to enable a fair and reliable assessment.
- SP practitioners (individuals who train SPs for assessments) need to understand principles of assessment.
- There are several phases in the preparation of SPs for assessments that involve cognitive and behavioural elements for repeated, standardized portrayal.
- Principles of deliberate practice apply to the attainment of 'assessment readiness' by individual SPs.
- After assessments, obtaining feedback from SPs, reviewing taped encounters and debriefing SPs are valuable practices for quality improvement.

OVERVIEW

Performance assessment in health professions education, training and certification has embraced human and non-human simulation as context to permit the development and assessment of behavioural, technical and problem-solving skills, as a proxy for real life. Simulation allows learning and assessment 'on demand', standardization of the content and the assessment criteria and customization for expected learning outcomes. For assessment purposes, particularly when high-stakes decisions are made on the basis of the assessment, consistent and standardized case presentation facilitates greater reliability and validity in the assessment process, feedback provided and decisions regarding mastery or qualifications. This chapter explores the concepts and methods of deliberate practice and quality assurance in standardizing SP performance and the criteria for determining the 'assessment readiness' of SPs, when repeating the portrayal for multiple learners by one SP at one site or involving multiple SPs and trainers in multiple sites, on multiple occasions.

Introduction

This chapter documents scholarly and practical approaches to SP methodology in assessments. Because SPs are the 'examination questions' in performance-based assessments, SP practitioners must appreciate principles of assessment, particularly related to the training of SPs and how they translate into high-quality SP-based assessments. We discuss key aspects of SP portrayal for assessment, including standardization. Roles and responsibilities of SPs are outlined and the SP as assessor is considered.

Simulated Patient Methodology: Theory, Evidence and Practice, First Edition. Edited by Debra Nestel and Margaret Bearman.
© 2015 John Wiley & Sons, Ltd. Published 2015 by John Wiley & Sons, Ltd.

The role of SPs in assessments

SPs play an integral role in assessment in many health education contexts(1–3). They are often described in an objectified manner as 'items', 'tools' or 'instruments' that are 'used'(4,5). In fact, SPs are crucial co-participants in an assessment, working as human 'examination questions' or proxies for real patients, at the centre of the care that learners are expected to demonstrate(5,6).

SPs are well suited to graded assessments of performance when judgements are required of a learner's ability to communicate and educate, to observe and evaluate and to adapt to patient (or client) needs. Further, SPs are suited when these judgements need to be made for many learners in a comparable way(7,8).

Typically in SP-based assessments, learners move through a circuit of stations (or scenarios), demonstrating their skills via interactions with SPs. Scenarios can include history taking, performing physical examinations, counselling, planning the management of patient care, collaborating with other health professionals and undertaking specific communication challenges (e.g. breaking bad news, ethical dilemmas) (see Chapter 2). Procedural skills may be assessed through hybrid simulation, in which an SP is aligned with another simulator (e.g. task trainer). Either an observing clinician assessor or the SP judges the learner's performance by completing a scoring tool, and/or by providing oral or written feedback.

Assessment-related terms

Various multi-station assessment formats with SPs have been developed. The *objective structured clinical examination (OSCE)* consists of a number of stations (usually 5–10 minutes long) with focused instructions. The less structured *clinical practice examination (CPX)* features longer stations (15–50 minutes) where learners interact with a patient as they might do in real practice and then write a post-encounter patient note(2,3,9,10).

Within these various formats, there are two main types of assessment. *Formative* assessments are intended to support learners during a period of study in advancing their skills and therefore must include some form of progress measure over a period of study and feedback. These are sometimes referred to as 'ungraded' assessments. *Summative* assessments are always 'graded' and evaluate a learner's achievement mastery following a period of study and may determine if a learner is ready for the next level of study. *High-stakes assessment* is a type of summative assessment that includes decisions such as passing to the next level of study, certification and licensure. Learners in high-stakes assessments are often referred to as candidates, so hereafter we use this term. Although SPs in summative contexts are often referred to as *standardized*, we continue to use the term simulated patient (SP) as the person whose behaviour is *standardized* for the purpose of assessment.

The development of SP methodology for assessment

Over the last 50 years, several drivers or attempts to advance measurement of performance or competence have influenced the development of SP methodology for assessment(1,9,11). In the 1960s, there was a movement away from 'knowledge' to 'performance' discourse, in which candidates demonstrated a more comprehensive scope of their competence through behaviour in either real or simulated scenarios and were evaluated by an observer(11). During this time, SPs were introduced into medical education(11–13). By the 1980s, 'psychometric' discourse emerged and aimed to 'represent human characteristics and behaviours with numbers for comparison purposes'(11). Systematic and standardized processes, related to all aspects of the assessment design, were introduced, to allow for effective statistical analysis and to control variance(11). Millman and Greene noted that 'a standardized test is one for which the conditions of administration and the scoring procedures are designed to be the same in all uses of the test. The conditions of administration include the physical test setting, the directions to examinees, the test materials and the time factors.'(14, p. 340). Presenting essentially the same context and stimuli enables candidates to demonstrate the competencies being tested. Reflecting this movement, SPs were renamed *standardized patients*(15).

By the 1990s, 'production' discourse arose, coinciding with the increasing emergence of national, distributed high-stakes SP-based assessments.

There was an even greater emphasis on the delivery of standardized outcomes in all aspects of the assessment through the implementation of rigorous quality assurance practices(11). *Performance*, *standardization* and *quality assurance* concepts derived from these discourses, are foundational principles of SP assessment methodology.

SP performance for assessment

SPs must holistically embody all aspects of the person they are representing, fluidly synthesizing cognitive, affective and psychomotor domains, to present an authentic portrayal, *as if* a real patient(1,16). They must memorize the *what*, specific given pieces of information contained in the scenario, and integrate this with the *how*, specific performance considerations (verbal and non-verbal behaviours, timing and quantity of information provided and affect presentation). They constantly have to negotiate and improvise (within the boundaries of the role and assessment protocols) through unscripted candidate approaches. They are simultaneously in and out of role, observing the encounter with a degree of detachment in order to provide appropriate specific stimuli (such as scripted lines and behaviours) and, where warranted, to retain and recall details in order to provide feedback and/or complete an assessment(16,17). They must perform as if naive, without being influenced by either their content knowledge of the role or biased by their interactions with other candidates. Actor training may be useful in some situations (e.g. high emotional affects), but is not a prerequisite, as the performance style of an SP is very different from that of an actor(1,10,16,18–20) (see Chapter 6).

Standardization of SP portrayal

A key aspect of SP portrayal for assessment is the principle of *standardization*, which refers to the consistency (reliability) and accuracy (validity) of their performance over time and between candidates so that each candidate is given the same fair and equal chance(3,21,22). Standardization can apply to an individual SP's portrayal or to SPs at the same or multiple sites, who are all portraying the same role and have been trained by the same or different SP practitioners. The higher the stakes,

the more rigorous is the need for standardization. However, what standardization looks like is not a universally agreed upon concept. At one end of the spectrum is the notion that all SPs doing the same role should have the same fixed external presentation, and at the other end is the assertion that, although all candidates must be presented with the same challenge, there will be variations in the portrayal of SPs doing the same role because each is a unique individual(1,15,16,23).

There is abundant psychometric research on SP-based assessments(7,24–30). It has been shown that portrayal of SPs can be standardized(7,31). However, variability occurs within and between SPs(27,31,32). Inconsistencies in SP performance (e.g. lack of appropriate cueing, withholding or providing misleading information, offering inaccurate physical findings or affect) impacts scores and issues arise from the selection and training of SPs and those who train them(22,31,33–36). This is not surprising, considering the diverse characteristics of SPs and faculty, including education, nature and amount of experience working in various assessment formats, exposure to SP methodology, flexibility, stamina and attitudes.

The training process

Training SPs for assessment performance is a nuanced and complex process, involving cognitive and behavioural elements. There is no accepted set of training standards and research related to SP training frequently lacks specific details and transparency. There are many descriptive accounts of contextually based training approaches(1–3,10,12,16,22,34–41).

The training process can be divided into four stages: preparation, training, session monitoring and continuous quality assurance and support. Training SPs to assess or give feedback will also be considered.

Stage 1 – preparation
Case and scoring tool development
Before training starts, cases and scoring tools, linked to objectives and competencies being tested, must be developed and piloted, often with the involvement of SP practitioners and SPs(2,3,10,36–40). Early and thorough role development and preparation are valuable quality assurance measures(27,38,40). However, there

is little documentation or research about this process(3).

Training resources

Training resources may include a *Training Guide*, *Assessment Readiness Form* and *training videos*(3,10,16,22,40,41). In the *Training Guide*, contextual details and key messages should be provided, including an explanation of assessment readiness and how it is achieved. Guidance should be given about the expected portrayal. Confidentiality, conflict of interest, examination security and procedures for dealing with errors should be addressed. Points of etiquette might include policies related to clothing, electronic devices, wearing of scented products, emergency evacuation and interacting with other SPs, candidates and assessors. An *Assessment Readiness Form* contains concrete, observable markers distilling key elements of the *Training Guide* and provides a transparent summary of the criteria that SPs need to perform in order to demonstrate assessment readiness. *Training videos* benchmarking SP performance are valuable, especially if the assessment is multi-site with several SP practitioners.

These tools provide context, expectations of roles, responsibilities and processes for SPs and SP practitioners and systematically frame and focus the process each time it occurs. Multi-site assessments especially benefit from these resources so that individuals across sites do not start to fill in perceived gaps or make assumptions about processes.

Recruiting SPs

Recruiting suitable SPs and SP practitioners is important to achieve quality and standardization of SP portrayal. Although little formal research has been done in this area, much has been written about appropriate qualities for SPs in assessment contexts(1,3,10,16,18,22,24,31,33,36,37,42). Considerations include demographic details of SPs (gender, age, physical characteristics), practical factors (availability, no conflict of interest, previous experience), skills (active listening, concentration, focus, attention to detail, ability to memorize), attitudes (openness to receiving feedback, flexibility, ability to reflect, professionalism, self-awareness of bias), intelligence and emotional stability. Having SPs play roles too closely aligned to their own experiences must be carefully considered to ensure this will not affect their ability to stay in role or their wellness. Not all SPs can do all kinds of assessments.

Stage 2 – training

Training sessions need to be carefully structured. In limited time, SP practitioners need to guide SPs to embody the role that they are portraying in a realistic, accurate and consistent manner. Although there are reports of SPs being handed a written role almost immediately before a summative assessment begins, this practice is unacceptable in terms of providing candidates a fair assessment. Drawing on principles of *deliberate practice*(43) is helpful to achieve *performance mastery* or assessment readiness through a recursive and repetitive process, involving targeted practice, rehearsal, performance and specific feedback(44,45).

There are several stages in preparing an SP for assessment (Figure 12.1). SPs new to assessments may need an orientation session, either in person and/or contained in the *Training Guide*. It is important to offer face-to-face training for all SPs performing the same role in order to introduce the SP role and scenario and the training video (if used) and to review assessment processes. Training all SPs doing the same role together ensures consistency and supports mutual benchmarking. Enabling the SP to review the role both individually and within the group can be beneficial. A variety of experiential, immersive, interactive training techniques that respond to

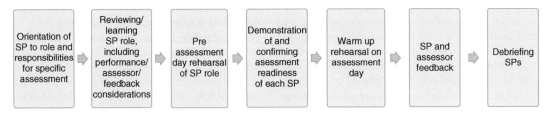

Figure 12.1 Training SPs for role portrayal in high-stakes assessments.

different learning preferences (e.g. auditory, visual, kinaesthetic) help SPs to embrace the performance function of their task and begin to embody the person they are portraying. A pre-examination day rehearsal or *dry run* where SPs demonstrate assessment readiness is very important(3,9,10,16,17,36,37,39,41). This phase may include clinicians, especially for a high-stakes assessment, who can role-play a range of candidates, allowing SPs to negotiate and improvise through unexpected candidate performances. An *Assessment Readiness Form* can be used as a precise 'diagnostic' tool to benchmark elements of an SP's performance, to formulate constructive feedback and to document readiness to participate in the assessment. Transparent procedures (e.g. further training, replacement) should be in place for SPs who are not assessment ready at the end of this phase(16,36,41).

Stage 3 – session monitoring

Briefing SPs immediately before the assessment orients them to logistics(38,40). A final rehearsal warms up the SP and the assessor and provides one more opportunity for ensuring standardization including appearance(33,41) (Figure 12.2). Monitoring and support throughout the assessment, through check-ins, direct observation (video, two-way mirror, in-room) and immediate attention to errors allow for timely support, adjustments and interventions(10,36,37,39). Debriefing SPs, immediately after the event, orally or in writing, helps to ensure their wellness and provides valuable feedback about roles and training information about candidate and assessor performance(1,3,10,16,18,21,37,41).

Stage 4 – continuous quality assurance

A common quality assurance method is post-assessment and analysis of actual interactions that were recorded during the assessment(2,27,36, 40,41). Trainers, SPs and quality assurance officers (Chief Examiner/Assessors) can review these recordings and make judgments about standardization.

SPs as assessors

In some contexts, SPs assess and/or provide feedback, even in high-stakes assessments. Evidence supports SPs in this role if they are rigorously trained to ensure consistency and accuracy and their assessment work is closely supervised(2,3,7,9,10,16,27,31,32,36,39,40,46–48). Training time must be significantly increased when SPs are both performing and assessing(1,3, 10,16,39). SPs must be taught to observe, interpret, recall and record their observations and/or to provide feedback according to a developed protocol(16). Scoring tools, filled in by hand or computerized, are usually one or some combination of checklists, rating scales or free text comments, capturing observations of specific behaviour and global impressions(2,3,9,10,16,28). Assessment criteria need clear benchmarking with specific anchors. Group discussions with all SPs scoring the same role are advised, including observing previous taped encounters to analyse, discuss, compare and come to inter-rater agreement about scoring(2,3,27).

Assessment criteria that SPs typically score relate to history taking, physical examination skills, interpersonal communication skills and spoken English proficiency(32,36,49). Evidence suggests that SPs can have similar accuracy to clinicians in these areas when using scoring tools, especially if the SP is only an observer rather than also being in role, but might be less effective in assessing more complex situations that reflect subtler aspects of clinical reasoning and expertise(7,9,27,46,48,50–54).

Benefits in having SPs assess are reported as including availability, cost-effectiveness, easiness to train and accuracy. Challenges include potential sources of error, hawk/dove tendencies, favouritism, carelessness, misinterpretation of the scoring tool, stereotyping, drift of scoring in reaction to candidate performances, personal biases, giving the candidate the benefit of the doubt, fatigue and inaccuracy of recall that occurs when assessing after the fact(2,3,7,10,12,16,27, 32,36,39,42,46,51,54). Newlin-Canzone et al. found that being an assessor and SP increases cognitive load and can affect an SP's ability to recall details accurately, especially related to non-verbal behaviour connected to unanticipated approaches not considered in training(17). Helping SPs to learn how to observe more closely, how to respond to diverse candidate approaches while in role (through the development of performance skills such as improvisation), raising their awareness of potential scoring errors and following up with quality assurance procedures (such as

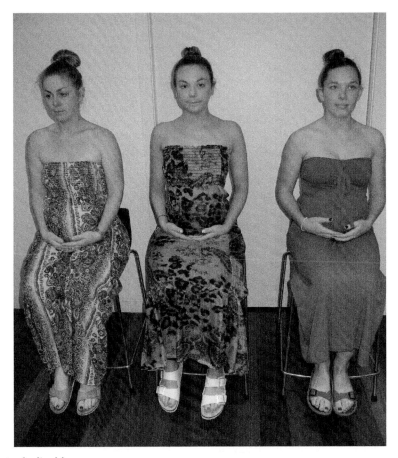

Figure 12.2 SPs standardized for appearance.

regularly scheduled reviews of taped encounters or refresher training) may be effective strategies for improving recall(17,27,31,40). It is important to note that SPs functioning in the role of assessor or giving feedback are not necessarily doing so from a patient perspective but rather as proxies for clinicians. Therefore, the focus of the SP assessment or feedback needs to be carefully considered and clearly framed.

Conclusion

SP methodology within assessment is highly influenced by the individual interpretations of all involved, making necessary explicit, strategic and rigorous training strategies that include attention to the portrayal style, the level of standardization and quality assurance processes.

Much of the published research and documentation is culturally biased. There are calls to test more complex situations involving interpersonal behaviour (e.g. collaboration, conflict resolution) and advanced procedural skills (in hybrid simulation) and to create ways to evaluate team performance(1,5,9,38,55). Calls for changes in assessment design, including ways to increase authenticity while balancing the need for standardization and creating opportunities to make more holistic, subjective (qualitative) judgements that move beyond psychometric and production discourses, will result in further evolution of SP methodology in assessment(23,29,55,56). Future research related to SP practitioners, training and other aspects of SP portrayal, including cultural influences, can provide further insight and inform practice(1,3,5,57). SP-based performance assessments continue to expand in scope, especially for high-stakes decisions(58). The creation of educational courses, formal standards of practice and national or international accreditation for SP practitioners and SPs will be important next steps in the evolution of SP methodology and assessment.

References

1 Cleland JA, Abe K and Rethans JJ (2009) The use of simulated patients in medical education: AMEE Guide No 42.1. *Medical Teacher*, **31**(6): 477–86.

2 Yudkowsky R (2009) Performance tests. In: Downing S and Yudkowsky R (eds) *Assessment in Health Professions Education*, pp. 217–43. Routledge, New York.

3 Howley LD (2013) Standardized patients. In: Levine AI, DeMaria S, Schwartz AD and Sim A (eds) *The Comprehensive Textbook of Healthcare Simulation*, pp. 173–90. Springer, New York.

4 Hodges BD (2007) A socio-historical study of the birth and adoption of the objective structured clinical examination (OSCE). Dissertation, University of Toronto.

5 Nestel D, Burn CL, Pritchard SA, Glastonbury R and Tabak D (2011) The use of simulated patients in medical education: Guide Supplement 42.1. Viewpoint. *Medical Teacher*, **33**(12): 1027–9.

6 Nestel D and Kneebone R (2010) Perspective: authentic patient perspectives in simulations for procedural and surgical skills. *Academic Medicine*, **85**(5): 889–93.

7 Van der Vleuten CP and Swanson DB (1990) Assessment of clinical skills with standardized patients: state of the art. *Teaching and Learning in Medicine*, **2**(2): 58–76.

8 Vu NV and Barrows HS (1994) Use of standardized patients in clinical assessments: recent developments and measurement findings. *Educational Researcher*, **23**(3): 23–30.

9 Boulet JR, Smee SM, Dillon GF and Gimpel JR (2009) The use of standardized patient assessments for certification and licensure decisions. *Simulation in Healthcare*, **4**(1): 35–42.

10 Zabar S, Kachur E, Kalet A and Hanley K (2013) *Objective Structured Clinical Examinations: 10 Steps to Planning and Implementing OSCEs and Other Standardized Patient Exercises*. Springer, New York.

11 Hodges B (2012) The shifting discourses of competence. In: Hodges B and Lingard L (eds) *The Question of Competence: Reconsidering Medical Education in the Twenty-First Century*, pp. 14–41. Cornell University Press, Ithaca, NY.

12 Barrows HS (1993) An overview of the uses of standardized patients for teaching and evaluating clinical skills. *AAMC. Academic Medicine*, **68**(6): 443–51.

13 Wallace P (1997) Following the threads of an innovation: the history of standardized patients in medical education. *Caduceus*, **13**(2): 5–28.

14 Millman J and Greene J (1993) The specification and development of tests of achievement and ability. In: Linn RF (ed.) *Educational Measurement*, 3rd edn, pp. 335–66. Macmillan, New York.

15 Norman GR, Tugwell P and Feightner JW (1982) A comparison of resident performance on real and simulated patients. *Academic Medicine*, **57**(9): 708–15.

16 Wallace P (2007) *Coaching Standardized Patients: for Use in the Assessment of Clinical Competence*. Springer, New York.

17 Newlin-Canzone ET, Scerbo MW, Gliva-Mcconvey G and Wallace AM (2013) The cognitive demands of standardized patients: understanding limitations in attention and working memory with the decoding of nonverbal behavior during improvisations. *Simulation in Healthcare*, **8**(4): 207–14.

18 McNaughton N, Tiberius R and Hodges B (1999) Effects of portraying psychologically and emotionally complex standardized patient roles. *Teaching and Learning in Medicine*, **11**(3): 135–41.

19 Nelles LJ (2011) My body, their story: performing medicine. *Canadian Theatre Review*, **146**(1): 55–60.

20 McNaughton NL (2012) A theoretical analysis of the field of human simulation and the role of emotion and affect in the work of standardized patients. Dissertation, University of Toronto.

21 Wallace J, Rao R and Haslam R (2002) Simulated patients and objective structured clinical examinations: review of their use in medical education. *Advances in Psychiatric Treatment*, **8**(5): 342–8.

22 Adamo G (2003) Simulated and standardized patients in OSCEs: achievements and challenges 1992–2003. *Medical Teacher*, **25**(3): 262–70.

23 Boulet JR (2012) Using SP-based assessments to make valid inferences concerning student abilities:pitfalls and challenges. *Medical Teacher*, **34**(9): 681–2.

24 Vu NV, Barrows HS, Marcy ML, Verhulst SJ, Colliver J and Travis T (1992) Six years of comprehensive, clinical, performance-based assessment using standardized patients at the Southern Illinois University School of Medicine. *Academic Medicine*, **67**(1): 42–50.

25 Hodges B, Regehr G, Hanson M and McNaughton N (1998) Validation of an objective structured clinical examination in psychiatry. *Academic Medicine*, **73**(8): 910–2.

26 Boulet JR, De Champlain AF and McKinley DW (2003) Setting defensible performance standards on OSCEs and standardized patient examinations. *Medical Teacher*, **25**(3): 245–9.

27 Boulet JR, McKinley DW, Whelan GP and Hambleton RK (2003) Quality assurance methods for performance-based assessments. *Advances in Health Sciences Education: Theory and Practice*, **8**(1): 27–47.

28 Boulet JR and Swanson DB (2004) Psychometric challenges of using simulations for high-stakes assessment. In: Dunn W (ed.) *Simulators in Critical Care Education and Beyond*, pp. 119–30. Society of Critical Care Medicine, Des Plaines, IL.

29 Howley LD (2004) Performance assessment in medical education: where we've been and where we're going. *Evaluation and the Health Professions*, **27**(3): 285–303.

30 Quero Munoz L, O'Byrne C, Pugsley J and Austin Z (2005) Reliability, validity and generalizability of an objective structured clinical examination (OSCE) for assessment of entry-to-practice in pharmacy. *Pharmacy Education*, **5**(1): 33–43.

31 Tamblyn RM, Klass D, Schnabl G and Kopelow M (1991) The accuracy of standardized patient presentation. *Medical Education*, **25**(2): 100–9.

32 Van Zanten M, Boulet JR and McKinley D (2007) Using standardized patients to assess the interpersonal skills of physicians: six years' experience with a high-stakes certification examination. *Health Commununication*, **22**(3): 195–205.

33 Tamblyn RM, Klass D, Schanbl G and Kopelow M (1990) Factors associated with the accuracy of standardized patient presentation. *Academic Medicine*, **65**(9): S55–6.

34 Beaulieu M, Rivard M, Hudon E, Saucier D, Remondin M and Favreau R (2003) Using standardized patients to measure professional performance of physicians. *International Journal for Quality in Heath Care*, **15**(3): 251–9.

35 Watson M, Norris P and Granas A (2006) A systematic review of the use of simulated patients and pharmacy practice research. *International Journal of Pharmacy Practice*, **14**(2): 83–93.

36 Furman GE (2008) The role of standardized patient and trainer training in quality assurance for a high-stakes clinical skills examination. *Kaohsiung Journal of Medical Sciences*, **24**(12): 651–5.

37 King AM, Perkowski-Rogers LC and Pohl HS (1994) Planning standardized patient programs: case development, patient training and costs. *Teaching and Learning in Medicine*, **6**(1): 6–14.

38 Smee S (2003) ABC of learning and teaching in medicine: skill based assessment. *BMJ*, **326**(7391): 703–6.

39 May W (2008) Training standardized patients for a high-stakes clinical performance examination in the California Consortium for the Assessment of Clinical Competence. *Kaohsiung Journal of Medical Sciences*, **24**(12): 640–5.

40 Furman GE, Smee S and Wilson C (2010) Quality assurance best practices for simulation-based examinations. *Simulation in Healthcare*, **5**(4): 226–31.

41 Smith C (2012) *SPs in Assessment (Module 7)*. www.vspn .edu.au (acsessed 13 September 2013).

42 Vu NV, Steward DE and Marcy M (1987) An assessment of the consistency and accuracy of standardized patients' simulations. *Journal of Medical Education*, **62**(12): 1000–2.

43 Ericsson KA, Krampe RT and Tesch-Römer C (1993) The role of deliberate practice in the acquisition of expert performance. *Psychological Review*, **100**(3): 363–406.

44 Wayne DB, Butter J, Siddall VJ, Fudala MJ, Wade LD, Feinglass J, et al. (2006) Mastery learning of advanced cardiac life support skills by internal medicine residents using simulation technology and deliberate practice. *Journal of General Internal Medicine*, **21**(3): 251–6.

45 Kneebone RL (2009) Practice, rehearsal and performance: an approach for simulation-based surgical and procedure training. *JAMA*, **302**(12): 1336–8.

46 Tamblyn RM, Klass DJ, Schnabl GK and Kopelow ML (1991) Sources of unreliability and bias in standardized-patient rating. *Teaching and Learning in Medicine*, **3**(2): 74–85.

47 Boulet JR, McKinley DW, Norcini JJ and Whelan GP (2002) Assessing the comparability of standardized patient and physician evaluations of clinical skills. *Advances in Health Sciences Education: Theory and Practice*, **7**(2): 85–97.

48 Vu N and Barrows H (1994) Use of standardized patients in clinical assessments: recent developments and measurement findings. *Educational Researcher*, **23**(3): 23–50.

49 Swanson DB, Norman GR and Linn RL (1995) Performance-based assessment: lessons from the health professions. *Educatioal Researcher*, **24**(5): 5–11.

50 Petrusa ER (2002) Clinical performance assessments. In: Norman G, Vleuten CM, Newble D, Dolmans DJM, Mann K, Rothman A, et al. (eds) *International Handbook of Research in Medical Education*, pp. 673–709. Springer, Dordrecht.

51 Vu NV, Marcy M, Colliver J, Verhulst S, Travis T and Barrows H (1992) Standardized (simulated) patients' accuracy in recording clinical performance check-list items. *Medical Education*, **26**(2): 99–104.

52 Colliver J and Williams R (1993) Technical issues: test application. AAMC. *Academic Medicine*, **68**(6): 454–60.

53 Quero-Munoz L, O'Byrne C and Pugsley J (2008) Impact of scoring method and examiner type on scores and outcomes in a national high-stakes pharmacy OSCE. Presented at the Ottawa Conference, 5–8 March 2008, Melbourne.

54 Turner JL and Dankoski ME (2008) Objective structured clinical exams: a critical review. *Family Medicine*, **40**(8): 574–8.

55 Hodges B (2013) Assessment in the post-psychometric era: learning to love the subjective and collective. *Medical Teacher*, **35**(7): 564–8.

56 Schuwirth L and Ash J (2013) Assessing tomorrow's learners: in competency-based education only a radically different holistic method of assessment will work. Six things we could forget. *Medical Teacher*, **35**(7): 555–9.

57 Howley L, Szauter K, Perkowski L, Clifton M and McNaughton N (2008) Quality of standardized patient research reports in the medical education literature: review and recommendations. *Medical Education*, **42**(4): 350–8.

58 McGaghie WC, Issenberg SB, Petrusa ER and Scalese RJ (2010) A critical review of simulation-based medical education research: 2003–2009. *Medical Education*, **44**(1): 50–63.

13 Simulated patient programme management

Tanya Tierney[1], Elaine E Gill[2] and Pamela J Harvey[3]

[1]Lee Kong Chian School of Medicine, Singapore
[2]King's College London Medical School at Guy's, King's and St Thomas' Hospitals, London, UK
[3]Monash University, Bendigo, Australia

 KEY MESSAGES

- Consider the needs of the organization in order to design the simulated patient (SP) programme appropriately.
- Careful recruitment and selection will ensure suitability of SPs.
- Ongoing professional development for SPs is crucial to maintain quality.

- Generic and scenario-specific training ensures that SPs will meet requirements; regular feedback supports individual development.
- Attention to the administrative aspects avoids problems associated with record keeping, communication and payment processing.

OVERVIEW

This chapter explores the administrative aspects of developing and maintaining a SP programme. It describes some of the important processes in starting and maintaining an SP programme, in addition to diverse approaches to recruitment and selection processes. Some of the logistical requirements are outlined, including choice of databases, modes of communication and payment factors. The key considerations of training and quality assurance of SP performance are discussed from a management perspective.

Introduction

SPs are an important part of the educational team and commitment to supporting the SPs will enhance the team as a whole. From a management perspective, bureaucratic supports include transparent and appropriate recruitment, selection and training processes, maintaining a database and working within a quality assurance framework. As part of this discussion, we also consider what administrative staffing is required and the potential of outsourcing to an SP agency. Some of the activities required are generally straightforward and can be supported by helpful advice from

administrators and finance without too much difficulty. It is also worth remembering that SPs can be talented and imaginative individuals who can be rich contributors to the overall educational programme and provide strong connections to the local community.

In some parts of the world, the profile of SP work is increasing as a professional career. In the United States, for example, some SPs work regularly enough to earn a living. In other places, it is still regarded as a casual arrangement with no formal career structure or path and SPs may take just occasional assignments. If SP work is more established, training and quality assurance

Simulated Patient Methodology: Theory, Evidence and Practice, First Edition. Edited by Debra Nestel and Margaret Bearman.
© 2015 John Wiley & Sons, Ltd. Published 2015 by John Wiley & Sons, Ltd.

practices also tend to be more consistent. This chapter draws from different traditions of SP management to describe good practices regarding the administrative aspects of working with SPs.

Starting a new programme

Developing an SP programme from scratch can seem like a big challenge and it is worth asking some key questions first. They include the following:

- *What is the level of institutional support, engagement and funding available?*
  If the institute is unfamiliar with the benefits of SPs within an educational team then pedagogical evidence may be required. An outline proposal can document the programme plan, including aims, administrative and management costs and potential outcomes. This can then be used to frame the discussion, rather than a more general request(1).
- *Why is an SP programme needed?*
  For example, if there are specific requirements for curricular activities or assessments, these can affect how the programme is developed.
- *What is the vision for the SP programme?*
  This may differ from the immediate institutional needs. Thinking more broadly and taking a 'blue sky' approach can ensure that the programme is not driven purely by administrative requirements such as examinations, but can work innovatively to improve the learning environment or support research initiatives.
- *Is there an existing local SP community?*
  If there are several institutions relatively close together, there can be benefits both for the institutions and the SPs themselves in working collaboratively. Exploring collaboration can be very valuable for all aspects of SP programme management.

Recruitment and selection of SPs

In general, there are two main avenues for recruiting SPs – from the community (lay performers) or accessing trained actors. Less commonly, but sometimes necessarily, health professionals can be considered, particularly if they have had SP training and are part of the programme faculty. Recruitment will depend on the required SP activities and the complexity of these roles. When planning recruitment, be clear on the desired SP qualities, in order to advertise strategically. If there is an existing SP community in close proximity then advertising can be relatively straightforward. Neighbouring institutions (such as hospitals or higher education institutions) may help make contact with SPs who work for them and formal collaborative arrangements may be very valuable.

If the programme requires lay people from the general community, patient involvement groups or charity groups such as Rotary, Lions or the YMCA may be good places to start. Many of these groups are looking for guest speakers and talking about the training of health professional students is a good way to engage. Community members who become SPs often do so because they feel that they are assisting in the training and development of their health professional workforce. Careful selection processes are necessary and SP motivation needs to be considered so that sessions are not used as an opportunity to focus on negative healthcare experiences. It is important to remember that even simple roles have a degree of SP decision-making in them(2), depending on how students ask questions or react to the scenario. Every SP needs careful training.

For complex roles, there is much discussion about the need for SPs to have a formal acting background. This may depend on what activities the SPs will be participating in. For example, if highly emotional roles are required, the need for acting skills may be higher than if the roles are less challenging. Similarly, acting skills are beneficial if SPs have to: play multiple roles; be able to step into and out of role quickly; or to change aspects of the scenario with direction from the facilitator. If recruiting actors, advertising should be targeted at places where actors are trained, such as theatre groups, acting schools or drama departments at schools.

When recruiting, it is also important to consider the demographics of the SP roles. Do SPs need to be a specific gender, age or ethnicity? It is common in SP programmes to find that minority groups and younger SPs are under-represented, so again targeting specific groups may be helpful. Having a broad range of SPs available to be involved increases the programme's capacity to enhance scenarios by ensuring that the SPs hired for particular scenarios are credible with respect to gender, age, weight and so on(3).

Many medical schools involving SPs will have a web page outlining what an SP does and how to apply. This can form the main conduit for information dissemination. A Frequently Asked Questions (FAQ) page is useful and a direct link to an application form can streamline the application process. The form could be a downloadable pdf or word processing document or an online form that feeds directly into a database. When designing the application form, consider what information, including demographic details, is needed for matching SPs to any proposed activities. Application forms should include a statement about privacy and where the SP information is kept, and some institutions have their application forms checked by their legal team before general distribution. An example application form is shown in Figure 13.1.

Once recruited, SPs must be selected, as not all applicants will be suitable. Selection processes depend on many factors – it is easy to be more selective if oversubscribed than if there are too few applicants. When selecting, again consider the programme's requirements. For example, if SPs are required to give detailed verbal feedback then their capacity to provide feedback should be taken into account.

If many people are being recruited at the same time, inviting potential participants to a group session is more time efficient than one-to-one interviews. A group session can start with a presentation about the programme and what qualities are desirable. This could be followed by some practical activities around scenario performance and giving feedback. Be aware that the more SPs who attend the session, the less is learnt about each attendee. The impact of a large number of SPs can be mitigated by increasing the number of facilitators. A decision to include each applicant in the programme can be made after the initial training session and applicants may withdraw once they realize what the programme entails.

SP databases

An organized and well-maintained database is crucial to the effective management of an SP programme. There are three main considerations in choosing a database. First, consider what information is to be recorded. Even the application form details and the initial selection interview or audition generate a lot of data regarding each SP.

Second, consider the available funds and resources such as administrative support. Funding should include a budget for maintenance of the database – many programmes do an annual review of the SPs on their list. Finally, consider the potential of an automated system, which allows SPs to update their own information online or have reminder emails and pay forms automatically generated by a system.

There are many software options for SP databases. The simplest (and probably the most commonly used), is a spreadsheet software package. While this is good for storing contact details and demographics, scope can be limited (for example, it may be difficult to store photographs). In addition, the programme might wish to retain a record of the activities performed by the SPs, e.g. teaching sessions, objective structured clinical examinations (OSCEs), scenarios and student encounters. Some institutions create their own database software depending on their particular needs. This is useful for a larger SP programme that is shared over many sites. There are also commercially available SP databases in packages that can link with video recordings of encounters.

Generic simulation management software solutions may have scope to include SP databases. These are often extensive large-scale simulation software packages, which include the need to record and review simulations (both SP and manikin) and manage the associated data. These large packages treat SP data as a simulation 'inventory item', so the SP database is a small part of the package. Large packages with extensive functionality are often not cost-effective for smaller programmes.

Training and quality assurance

Training can be generic to the overall programme or specific to a role. It helps SPs in the understanding of their roles if they are fully briefed on the aims of the overall health professional training course and understand their involvement in the 'big picture'. This can form a starting point when designing generic training. Training sessions can emphasize the professional standards expected from the SPs, such as punctuality, commitment and communication with SP programme staff. It also should outline the rights of the SP, as an employee. It is helpful to think of training SPs as

PERSONAL PARTICULARS					
Full Name (underline Family Name): Preferred name:			Home / Postal Address:		
Gender:	Ethnicity:		(Home Contact)		(Mobile Contact)
Nationality:	Country of Birth:		Email Address		
Date of Birth (dd/mm/yyyy):			(Emergency Contact Name & No.)		

PHYSICAL CHARACTERISTICS (please tell us about any scars, piercings, tattoos or other physical characteristics)

Height (m)	Weight (kg)	Role playing age range

LANGUAGE PROFICIENCY (Please state languages and proficiency level, i.e. excellent, good, fair, poor)

Spoken:	
Written:	

RELEVANT MEDICAL HISTORY (please tell us about any medical conditions you have or past medical history that may be relevant to your work as an SP).

RELEVANT EXPERIENCE IN ACTING / ROLE PLAY / SP WORK

Figure 13.1 Example application form for simulated patient.

OTHER RELEVANT SKILLS (e.g. teaching, sign language, etc.)

REASON FOR INTEREST IN SP WORK (Brief description)

ARE YOU WILLING TO TAKE PART IN PHYSICAL EXAMINATION SESSIONS (Y/N)
(Please elaborate if you want to specify)

Where did you hear about the SP programme?

Kindly submit this form together with two photos (one full length and
one head and shoulders) to SPadmin@organisation

Figure 13.1 (*Continued*)

a form of professional development. If SPs also work in other SP programmes or in other sectors such as corporate role play, training may benefit their other activities. Likewise, any training they receive in other sectors may benefit their SP work.

When training, SPs' backgrounds must be taken into account. For example, working with professional actors means less focus on acting/role-play skills. If SPs are required to give feedback, it is important to include comprehensive feedback skills in the generic training(4). Trained actors are not necessarily more skilled at this than non-actors. When training SPs for feedback, consider how to train SPs to step in and out of three different positions in each session: (a) the character and attached health problems; (b) observing and logging the learner's responses and communication behaviours; and (c) offering feedback on these in a way that is useful for the learner. We would recommend including SP feedback for learners where possible to maximize the educational value of the session (see Chapter 10 for more details).

Most SPs are also given specific training sessions relating to particular assignments. This is especially important if standardized performance is expected for high-stakes assessments(5). An in-depth discussion on SP training and SPs in assessment can be found in Chapters 9 and 12, respectively.

Educating SP trainers and facilitators is a major issue and is labour intensive. There may be courses available but often programmes must develop their own SP trainer/facilitator professional development. Remember to build this into programme design and costing and consider any required payments. There are resources available from various institutions to help design basic SP trainer/facilitator courses(6). If starting a new programme and recruiting rapidly, training sessions may include relatively large numbers of SPs. As with the recruitment auditions, keep in mind the ratio of SP trainers to SPs.

Quality assurance of SP performance can be a problematic area and is sometimes neglected in SP programmes. Often underperforming SPs are identified by informal feedback and SPs are dropped from a programme without communication. That is, they are simply not called again for assignments once identified as underperforming. This is easily done as SP work is often by invitation to one assignment at a time. However,

as educators, we stress to SPs the importance of feedback to students as part of their professional development, so it is good practice also to let SPs know that they should expect to receive feedback on their performance(1). In this way, SPs will not be surprised if they are observed as part of quality assurance or feedback is provided by SP facilitators. The programme faculty, SP facilitators and SPs should have a clear idea of what SP performance indicators are and how these are measured. Some questions to think about are:

- Will there be specific observations of their performance? Will ongoing feedback be provided by others (e.g. SP facilitators/students)?
- Can the SPs be observed remotely (e.g. from a control room) or does an observer need to be present?
- Will feedback be supported by a particular instrument/form assessing SP performance (see Figure 13.2 for an example of a form designed for this) or will feedback/assessment be purely through commentary?
- How will goals be set for improvement in response to feedback?
- What behaviours would prompt discontinuation of the involvement of a particular SP? How might this be communicated to the SP?

The availability of SPs will also determine performance standards; an oversubscribed programme can afford to be discriminating. A quality assurance check may also be an effective way of recording the most suitable roles for specific SPs in the programme database.

Communication with SPs

Communication with SPs is dependent on both their needs and the programme requirements. Emailing is efficient but there may be individuals in the programme who do not have access to email. In this instance, alternative arrangements such as communication by telephone may be required. Consider the convenience of text message reminders as an alternative to email reminders.

Communication can help maintain relationships with the SPs, such as thank-you emails after an assignment or feedback on performance. If there is a relatively large pool of SPs who are infrequently involved, it may be worth thinking about additional modes of communication. A regular

SP Name:		Role:			Student:		

Domain	Not done / well below expectation	Below expectation	Borderline	Meets expectation	Above expectation	Well above expectation
Response to student behaviours	0	1	2	3	4	5
Accuracy of information given	0	1	2	3	4	5
Accuracy of non-verbal behaviours	0	1	2	3	4	5
Overall realism of role-play	0	1	2	3	4	5
Appropriate positive feedback	0	1	2	3	4	5
Appropriate developmental feedback	0	1	2	3	4	5
Wording and specificity of feedback	0	1	2	3	4	5
Overall quality of verbal feedback	0	1	2	3	4	5
Appropriate Likert scale feedback	0	1	2	3	4	5
Appropriate written comments	0	1	2	3	4	5

Something that was done well

Suggestions for improvement

Any other comments

Figure 13.2 Example rating form for SP performance.

newsletter can help them feel connected and also keep them updated about the organization as a whole. An end-of-year celebration for SPs may be another way of thanking them for their work and checking whether they would like to continue their participation.

Payments and funding models

Payment to SPs will be influenced by institutional policy and by relevant employment laws. Comparisons of different programmes reveal many ways in which this is done(7). In some institutions, SPs are considered to be casual employees who are paid by the hour/session at particular award rates. In others, they may have more formal appointments and hold a fixed, part-time position. Payment issues can be complex, so liaise with Human Resources and Finance departments to discuss processes. It is worth considering the following questions:

- Are contracts or formal paperwork required?
- Does tax or other payments need to be paid on the SP's behalf?
- What declarations are required by the SPs regarding tax?
- What employment conditions such as protected breaks per given number of hours are required?
- What, if any, are the annual leave allowances or additional pay equivalents?

Creating documentation around reimbursement is useful for new staff members. Documentation, accounting and rates of pay should be transparent to protect the programme, the institution and the SPs. Prompt payment is always appreciated.

One of the important decisions for any SP programme is how much to pay. If there is a local 'going rate' this can provide guidance, but consideration should be given as to whether a fixed pay rate is appropriate or if there should be different rates for different assignments. Some institutions pay more for performances that need higher skills levels, such as:

- highly emotional scenarios;
- psychiatric illness portrayals;
- roles involved in making films for teaching purposes.

Some institutions pay different rates for:

- physical examination assignments – there are examples of those who pay more on the basis that portrayal of physical signs is a highly skilled role and others who pay less on the basis that it is a 'non-speaking role';
- teaching, assessment or a research project assignments;
- providing feedback to learners;
- quality of performance, such as realism of role-play, ability to play high challenge roles or quality of feedback.

One advantage of a graduated pay scale is that it can increase buy-in for the quality assurance process as there is perceived benefit for high performance. It is helpful to define clearly the criteria for the different rates of pay to ensure transparency and avoid potential conflict.

Some SP programmes work with volunteers. People engage in SP work for various reasons and there are many successful SP programmes that involve volunteers. Volunteer SPs need to have the same understanding of the programme as paid SPs and therefore should undertake the same selection process and training to maintain quality assurance. Consider other ways of demonstrating how much volunteer input is valued, such as paying travel expenses, catering or emails showing appreciation. Thank-you cards signed by the students can reinforce the value of the volunteer work.

SP programme staffing

SP programmes vary in size. Some are small and can be coordinated by a single person as part of their role. Others are large and have several dedicated staff. The requirements of roles within programmes may differ between institutions. Questions to consider in staffing are:

- Is a dedicated administrator required to manage the SP programme?
- Could this role be combined with a related role (e.g. OSCE administrator or Communication Skills teaching administrator?).
- How many staff members are needed, based on the size of the programme?
- Will teaching faculty, clinicians or SPs be SP trainers?
- Is a dedicated SP trainer required?

There are an increasing number of commercial SP agencies, so outsourcing some of the SP programme to an agency is an option. If the programme works with an agency, it often streamlines recruitment, training and payment processes, which in turn may reduce staff numbers and workload issues. There are also additional benefits, such as a replacement SP when there is illness, for example. The cost per session will be greater but this can be offset by the programme's own reduction in staff overheads. Good communication is needed with the agency to clarify what the programme's needs are in order to ensure appropriate SPs for the assignments. The limitations of working with an agency are less control over training, selecting and building relationships with individual SPs.

Conclusion

There are many considerations when setting up and maintaining an SP programme. Clarity is required about the aims of the programme and the scope of practice for SPs, keeping in mind the available institutional support and funding. Effective advertising that targets the correct people, careful selection and initial training will provide a good start to building a pool of SPs. Clear terms and agreement, governance and quality processes, coupled with ongoing training and development, will help maintain high standards and ensure that the SP programme continues to meet the educational needs of the institution.

References

1 Ker JS, Dowie A, Dowell J, Dewar G, Dent JA, Ramsay J, *et al.* (2005) Twelve tips for developing and maintaning a simulated patient bank. *Medical Teacher*, **27**(10): 4–9.
2 Harvey P and Radomski N (2011) Performance pressure: simulated patients and high-stakes examinations in a regional clinical school. *Australian Journal of Rural Health*, **19**(6): 284–9.
3 Cleland JA, Abe K and Rethans J (2009) The use of simulated patients in medical education: AMEE Guide No 42. *MedicalTeacher*, **31**(6): 477–86.
4 Bokken L, Linssen T, Scherpbier A, van der Vleuten C and Rethans J (2009) Feedback by simulated patients in undergraduate medical education: a systematic review of the literature. *Medical Education*, **43**(3): 202–10.
5 Adamo G (2003) Simulated and standardized patients in OSCEs: achievements and challenges 1992–2003. *Medical Teacher*, **25**(3): 262–70.
6 Monash University (2014) *Teaching Resources*. http://www.med.monash.edu.au/srh/learning-teaching/resources.html (accessed 7 July 2014).
7 Nestel D, Tabak D, Tierney T, Layat-Burn C, Robb A, Clark S, *et al.* (2011) Key challenges in simulated patient programs: an international comparative case study. *BMC Medical Education*, **11**: 69.

Part 4

Case Studies: Innovations Across the Health Professions

14 Real patient participation in simulation

Rosamund Snow

King's Health Partners, London, UK

OVERVIEW

In standard simulations, there is an assumption that real patients would choose the same learning outcomes and responses as medical educators and actors do. This is not always appropriate, particularly when dealing with people who have long-term or incurable conditions, where the majority of healthcare work is done by patients themselves. In 'patient-driven simulation', these assumptions are challenged. A project was devised in which people with Type 1 diabetes designed, wrote, delivered and led feedback on a series of successful simulation scenarios. Patient educators prioritised a different curriculum from that chosen by their medical colleagues, including an emphasis on learning how to switch back and forth between communication and technical skills, the need to interact with the patient as part of the healthcare team and resilience in handling ambiguous situations. In feedback, students praised the patient-driven model as closer to real life than standard simulation.

Rationale

Modern simulated learning creates remarkably realistic scenarios in terms of setting and student experience, but one thing is usually missing – real patients.

When no real patients are involved, two major assumptions are made: first, that actors and the educators who brief them can really simulate patients – that they know how real patients would respond in a given scenario; second, that learning outcomes set by healthcare personnel are the most appropriate for the situation – that real patients would want students to learn those things.

In chronic disease, which is on the rise, this issue is of particular importance. Caring for patients with chronic conditions is very different from the traditional patient–doctor model of care; the modern doctor or nurse increasingly needs a skill-set oriented around chronic support rather than acute treatment(1). It is sometimes argued that most simulated patients (SPs) and simulation educators will have some personal experience of being a patient and interacting with healthcare professionals in their ordinary lives, and can bring that to bear when creating a simulation scenario. However, living with a long-term condition is a qualitatively different experience from a one-off diagnosis and course of treatment. An illness that must be managed rather than cured brings with it specific psychological issues, in addition to the prospect of a lifetime of interactions with health services. In contrast to the traditional acute patient, most healthcare work associated with chronic disease is done by the layperson with that disease, as part of ordinary life, and they may know more about managing their condition than the professionals they come into contact with(2).

In healthcare education, patient stories, complaints and experiences have been used in a variety of ways, particularly to teach communication skills, but the patient voice continues to be filtered through clinicians' perspectives(3). It is still rare for patients to be involved in writing scenarios, setting learning outcomes and giving feedback, although where it has been tried, there have been clear differences between the priorities

Simulated Patient Methodology: Theory, Evidence and Practice, First Edition. Edited by Debra Nestel and Margaret Bearman.
© 2015 John Wiley & Sons, Ltd. Published 2015 by John Wiley & Sons, Ltd.

Table 14.1 Programme overview.

Overall aim	To include genuinely patient-driven learning outcomes for healthcare professionals in simulation scenarios
Learning objectives	1. Understand the long-term impact on the patient of good/poor communication and learn how to adapt communication to the patient
	2. Practice combining good clinical skills with good communication, rather than doing one and then the other
	3. Consider how to react to ambiguous situations where preset protocols may not be appropriate
	4. Learn how to operate alongside patients with chronic conditions as part of the healthcare team
	5. Explore how to manage the emotions and challenges inherent in caring for a patient who has more disease-specific knowledge than the healthcare professional
Target participants	Available to all healthcare professionals, pre- and post-graduation. Two students at a time can participate directly in each simulation scenario, with up to 10 observing and actively taking part in debrief and feedback sessions
Setting	Emergency Room ward in dedicated Simulation Centre
Program/Session length	Two or three patient-driven scenarios normally combined with a further two or three clinician-driven scenarios to deliver a full day's training (five sessions in all)
Faculty	1–2 medical faculty with several years' experience, 3 patient faculty, initially with no experience
Simulator(s)	Mixture of real patients as SPs, SPs briefed by patients and manikins voiced by patients
Frequency of offering	Although patient-driven scenarios can be run without the presence of patients, feedback suggests that the full benefit comes from debriefing sessions with real patient involvement. This is therefore dependent on patient availability

identified by real patients, as opposed to those assumed by SPs(4,5).

This case study draws on a collaboration between clinicians and patients with chronic disease in which the patients genuinely drove the project. As a researcher with a long-term condition, I was supported by a medical and administrative team to create, with an Advisory Group of fellow patients, an educational intervention informed entirely by outcomes that people with chronic conditions had chosen for students to learn. The simulation scenarios and learning points were conceived, designed, delivered, written and evaluated by patients, with minimal intervention by clinicians.

Scenario example

Setting

The project setting was the Simulation and Interactive Learning Centre (SAIL) at St Thomas' Hospital in London (http://www.guysandstthomas .nhs.uk/education-and-training/sail/simulation -and-interactive-learning-centre.aspx). This high-fidelity centre runs regular training for pre- and post-qualification healthcare staff across disciplines, working with SPs and manikins in a range of settings from multi-bed simulated wards to

outreach primary care settings. Learners have a chance to work together to solve problems in preset scenarios and then work with their peers and simulation educators to share feedback and reflections on the experience. An overview is presented in Table 14.1.

Creating patient-driven simulation

The patient-driven project used the same facilities and format as an ordinary simulation, but preparation for it differed from the standard procedures in several ways. No clinicians were involved in collecting or interpreting patient experiences. Instead, as a layperson with Type 1 diabetes, I recruited 15 others from an online diabetes community to an Advisory Group, to discuss the learning outcomes they wanted to prioritize based on their combined 400 years of living with a chronic illness. Three of us worked with the centre's simulation experts to turn these into workable scenarios that could be run in the SAIL Emergency Room wards and then acted as 'patient educators'. In this role, we oversaw the learning and directed our own involvement. We briefed the SPs, used our own voices for manikins or became SPs ourselves in the 'patient' role in scenarios. In briefing others, we were able to describe physical and emotional processes from our own lived experience, creating a more accurate simulation; because the patient simulators wore earpieces throughout, we were able to direct their responses as the scenario unfolded. This also had the advantage of providing a valuable emotional buffer between real patient and student. Watching an SP act out a threatening or upsetting situation was less demanding than attempting to relive it ourselves.

The 'medic educators' offered administrative support, translation of medical jargon and procedures and advice on teaching technique. Owing to their far greater experience in running simulation training, the medical educators led structured feedback sessions at first, requesting patient participants' perspectives; they then stepped back as the patient educators gained confidence and led post-simulation feedback sessions. Patient-driven scenarios were interspersed with medic-driven ones as part of a full day's training in the SAIL Centre. Standard evaluation forms, with a mixture of closed and open questions about the experience, were used to gather feedback from learners; the participants were a mixture of pre- and post-qualification healthcare professionals from a variety of disciplines. A sample scenario can be seen in Box 14.1.

In evaluation, learners were enthusiastic about several key aspects of patient-driven simulation. In particular, they felt that the element of ambiguity made the scenarios 'a lot more real' than those where there was a preferred course of action. They also enjoyed the opportunity to interact with the patient educators during feedback, specifying that the key learning points of the day arose from this discussion. Patient educators described the project as 'radical'; unlike other patient involvement initiatives we had experienced, we felt we had been genuinely listened to. However, the emotional toll of recreating situations with echoes from our own lives was surprisingly high for some of us, particularly those who had taken part as SPs or as the voice of the manikin. As unpaid volunteers, we were also absorbing the financial and time cost of days off work and study, a situation that could not continue indefinitely.

Key messages

There were qualitative differences between patient educators' priorities and those set by the medical educators. Clinician-driven outcomes emphasized

such things as clear communication, handover skills, teamwork amongst healthcare staff, the importance of knowing when to call for help and the use of specific protocols and pathways. Patient-driven outcomes focused on teaching students not only how to communicate, but also how to switch back and forth between communication and technical skills; teamwork that included the patient in addition to other staff; and how to handle ambiguous situations that have no clear pathway.

Lessons learnt

- *DO* ask patients to set learning outcomes; what they prioritize and emphasize may surprise you and create better teaching environments.
  DO NOT ask patients to help unless you are prepared to listen and perhaps have your assumptions challenged.

- *DO* get a layperson, ideally a patient, to collate other patients' responses and translate them into workable learning outcomes.
  DO NOT filter patients' suggestions through clinicians to fit a pre-existing set of learning outcomes.

- *DO* consider what will happen if you do not agree with the patient-driven learning outcomes. For example, raise the issue in feedback so students appreciate where the medical worldview may clash with patients' worldview and discuss how they might handle it in practice.
  DO NOT discard patient-driven outcomes because they don't fit hospital protocol or your textbook teaching.

- *DO* allow patient educators time beforehand to discuss how they will turn their own experiences and emotions into constructive learning for students in the debrief.
  DO NOT ignore or silence patients who feel upset and angry as a result of past healthcare interactions. Their passion can be a key learning point for students.

- *DO* ensure the patient educators are supported, not overwhelmed by other educators, and able to hand over to others if simulation becomes too emotionally difficult.
  DO NOT have a 'token' patient surrounded by healthcare professionals or a set-up that has no Plan B if a patient needs to step back.

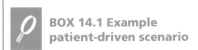

BOX 14.1 Example patient-driven scenario

Scenario: Hypoglycaemia co-morbidity

Summary: Patient played by an actor, briefed by the patient faculty. The patient is an adult male with a broken leg awaiting investigation by a specialist and therefore nil by mouth in case of potential surgery. He also has insulin-treated diabetes managed by two injections per day, meaning that without food at a set time, his blood sugar will go dangerously low. As his blood sugar drops, he becomes increasingly aggressive and paranoid and will not allow intravenous glucose to be administered.

Patient-driven learning outcomes:

1. Explore the boundaries between pragmatism and rules.
2. Consider the impact on the patient of having daily management decisions taken out of their hands.
3. Learn how to work with patients with chronic disease as part of the healthcare team.

Patient Role

Scenario

It is 12 noon on Tuesday morning. You were up early to start work on a new building site and had an accident in which you fell a short distance from some scaffolding and badly hurt your right foot. You were admitted to emergency at 9.00am, had X-rays relatively quickly and were told that your foot was broken and a further CT scan would be required.

You have been Type 1 diabetic since you were 5 years old and are on a twice-daily insulin regime. You take a mix of Humulin S and Humulin I at about 6.30am and around 5.30pm when you get home from work.

You have now been waiting 2½ hours and it's soon going to be the time you'd normally eat lunch. You know that if you don't eat soon you'll go hypo.

Underlying diagnosis

Hypoglycaemia

Patient instructions

At first you just ask whether it's possible to have some lunch or possible to leave soon.

Later you realise it's too late for a meal so you ask for your jacket, which is where you keep supplies of sugar and snacks.

You don't say the word hypo. You insist, 'I need my lunch', and as you start to feel sick and tingly, you say, 'I'm getting tingly in my lips now and my hands, I told you.'

You become more and more confused, aggressive and paranoid. After a few more minutes you say that you are feeling sweaty.

If anyone tries to give you intravenous glucose or injection of glucagon you become extremely angry – you don't trust what they are giving you. 'Why can't you just give me sugar, I'm not a vegetable, I can look after myself?'

If learners do find sugar or get you the jacket, you become rapidly less angry. Over 2–3 minutes you become quiet and calmer. By 5 minutes you are very apologetic.

If learners don't treat the hypo you become unconscious.

Patient faculty will brief you on physical symptoms and emotions of hypoglycaemia in this situation.

Comments

A recurrent theme across the Advisory Group's experiences was the frustration and fear caused when their self-management was overridden by hospital protocols, causing serious unwanted health outcomes. This scenario intentionally put students in a position where hospital procedures had broken down (nobody had discussed with the patient or planned how to manage his blood sugar over the lunchtime period), while at the same time a pragmatic response (to give the patient the Lucozade he requested) would mean that the student would have to 'break the rules' in terms of contravening the Registrar's orders on nil by mouth. The patient faculty also wanted to illustrate the importance of listening to the expertise offered by a person with chronic disease, who was initially clearly giving warnings about the consequences of a nil by mouth policy; in addition, the simulation aimed to get learners to consider the reasons behind the patient's anxiety at not being able to access medication (including foodstuffs) that he would normally have full responsibility for outside the hospital. Although this scenario was simple to run, it was the most difficult for students to handle, and created a great deal of passionate discussion in debrief.

- *DO* acknowledge the work being done by the patient educators, with financial reward or other incentive meaningful to them.

  DO NOT assume that the work the patient educators are doing is cheap. Many patients will offer their services without asking for anything in return, purely for the opportunity to make things better. Do not confuse this with low-value work or working for free.

References

1 WHO (2012) *Global Health Observatory Data Repository.* World Health Organization, Geneva.
2 Snow R, Sandall J and Humphrey C (2013) What happens when patients know more than their doctors? Experiences of health interactions after diabetes patient education: a qualitative patient-led study. *BMJ Open*, **3**(11): e003583.
3 Towle A, Bainbridge L, Godolphin W, Katz A, Kline C, Lown B, *et al.* (2010) Active patient involvement in the education of health professionals. *Medical Education*, **44**(1): 64–74.
4 Nestel D and Kneebone R (2010) Perspective: authentic patient perspectives in simulations for procedural and surgical skills. *Academic Medicine*, **85**(5): 889–93.
5 Nestel D, Cecchini M, Calandrini M, Chang L, Dutta R, Tierney T, *et al.* (2008) Real patient involvement in role development: evaluating patient focused resources for clinical procedural skills. *Medical Teacher*, **30**(5): 534–6.

15 Interprofessional community care: a simulated clinic for healthcare professional learners

Pamela J Taylor[1], Mollie Burley[1] and Debra Nestel[2]

[1]Monash University, Moe, Australia
[2]Monash University, Clayton, Australia

OVERVIEW

This case study describes an innovation in interprofessional social care in a rural community health service. It features simulated client roles drawn from real clients, volunteers recruited as simulated clients (SCs) and the criticality of strategic planning to obtain buy-in from staff at the health service.

Rationale

This case study describes an interprofessional simulated clinic based in a community setting in rural Victoria, Australia. Internationally, interest in interprofessional practice has been building following the recommendations of the World Health Organization(1) and several systematic reviews(2–5). The reviews identified the need for preparing health professionals for collaborative practice, for learning to work in teams and for developing services to improve care, including community health services. The reviews formed the basis of our evolving programme for entry-level healthcare professionals.

We sought to offer health professional learners on clinical placements in our community health service the opportunity to experience interprofessional collaboration. We aimed to establish interprofessional clinics as part of normal clinic practice, which would provide learners with an opportunity to 'learn with, from and about each other' to improve quality of patient care(6). However, we encountered many of the challenges documented with interprofessional education, such as scheduling learners from different disciplines (and institutions), clinical staff not being released to supervise and lack of familiarity with the concept of collaborative assessment and treatment(7).

In order to address these challenges, we used a stepwise approach. First, we sought 'buy in' from health service executive, healthcare practitioners (HCPs) and learners for the concept. This was addressed by introducing key executive and HCPs to concepts of interprofessional clinics. Monthly interprofessional workshops gave all learners on-site an opportunity to meet, learn about each other's scope of practice and participate in a paper-based simulation. At these sessions, learners formed small interprofessional teams and worked together to assess and prepare an interprofessional care plan for a simulated client (paper-based) with complex chronic conditions.

Having gained 'buy in', we progressed to establishing the simulated clinic. We needed to do the following:

- develop scenarios representing 'typical' community health clients with complex chronic health conditions;
- develop a protocol for a psychosocial screening interview, which could be used by any healthcare discipline;
- recruit and train simulated clients (SCs);
- schedule learners from up to 15 healthcare professions with the intersection of student placements at different times;
- enable observation of consultations through audio-visual recording;

Simulated Patient Methodology: Theory, Evidence and Practice, First Edition. Edited by Debra Nestel and Margaret Bearman.
© 2015 John Wiley & Sons, Ltd. Published 2015 by John Wiley & Sons, Ltd.

- minimize input from the already stretched HCPs;
- maintain relationships with HCPs by keeping them informed of developments.

Case study

We developed a SC training programme drawing on resources from the Victorian Simulated Patient Network (Table 15.1)(8). The learning objectives were that learners would be able to:

- collaborate with learners from a different healthcare profession;
- conduct a client-centred screening interview;
- complete a care plan for the client.

Development of scenarios

In order to develop scenarios that were authentic and relevant to community healthcare, we sought real stories from clients' initial contact at the Latrobe Community Health Service (LCHS). HCPs were asked to select eight clients with complex/chronic conditions that needed referral to several health services. A template was developed (MB) and these stories were entered into the template, noting salient issues which each client recounted at their initial visit. All personal identifiers were removed (Box 15.1).

Development of the Interprofessional Referral Tool

The Interprofessional Referral Tool (IRT) was developed by allied HCPs at LCHS. We needed a tool that could be used by clinicians from any profession with the purpose of providing a thorough bio-psycho-social screening to generate appropriate referrals to improve care of clients in the community with complex chronic conditions. The IRT covers medical history, mobility, social supports and emotional wellbeing, in addition to the ability to monitor and manage behaviour to benefit their own health. A care plan summary completes the tool.

Recruitment of simulated clients

Volunteers were recruited from the local community (Figure 15.1). Advertisements were placed in the local newspaper, volunteer newsletter and flyers at various LCHS sites in the region. The only requirements of SCs were that they were to have a good memory and be available to attend two training sessions. A $20 gift voucher was offered to assist volunteers with transport costs.

Training simulated clients

A 4 hour training session was developed for SCs – they were provided with a workbook with plain English explanations and visual prompts,

Table 15.1 Programme overview.

Aim	To develop a simulated clinic where health professional learners collaborated to screen simulated clients within the context and values of community health service
Learning objectives	After the session, the learners were expected to be able to: • collaborate with learners from different professions; • conduct a client-centred screening interview; • complete a care plan for the client
Target participants	Four to six learners were invited to each session. Learners from different professions worked in pairs to conduct a screening interview. The learners were from occupational therapy, physiotherapy, dietetics, speech pathology, art therapy, nursing, dentistry, medicine, paramedicine, community welfare, social work, counselling and psychology. Each session provided for a minimum of two learners with a maximum of four interviewing with capacity for an additional two student observers
Setting	The context for the simulation was a rural community health service, which emphasizes holistic client care within a psychosocial model of health. The simulated clinics were held on two sites in purpose-built consultation rooms
Session length	Each session lasted up to 4 hours and included two simulations. The session was structured with briefing, two interviews and debriefing (feedback)
Faculty	One interprofessional educator and one administrative/technical support person were required to run the session
Simulator	Simulated clients trained to portray authentic roles based on real clients in the local community Interviews were viewed live from another room via audio-visual link or through a one-way screen
Frequency	Learners had the opportunity to participate in two occasions during their placement

BOX 15.1 Simulated client role

Simulated Client Name   Ms Cherry Andrews, aged 30

Affects/Behaviours

- Feels depressed and hopeless
- Exacerbated by upcoming eviction – trouble paying arrears rent/private rental
- Needs public housing
- Worries for welfare of daughter

Presenting Problems

- Walks with a stick
- Requires food assistance
- Requires housing assistance
- Multiple sclerosis (MS)
- Severe anxiety

Social and Family History

- Early diagnosis of MS at age 25
- Soon after decided to have a child (daughter – Isabel, who is now aged 2)
- Living in Moe in rented property
- Experiencing difficulty with landlord over broken hot water service and worn carpets
- Tripped on frayed edge of carpet
- No hot showers
- Boils kettle for hot water
- Does not work
- Lives with partner – Shane
- Partner has a drinking problem contributing to financial problems
- Mother lives close by in a two-bedroom unit with other daughter (sister Kate) and grandchild
- Partner's family lives 20 km away
- Partner has casual work locally – receives carer allowance
- Partner helps with Isabel's care too
- No car at present
- Walks to community health service and other local amenities
- Mother occasionally looks after Isabel

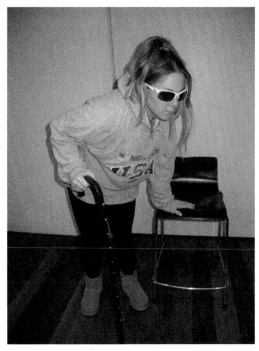

Figure 15.1 Image of simulated client.

recognizing that some volunteers came with a limited educational background. SCs were matched for age and appearance with a client story of their choosing from the eight that were developed. The training session focused on experiential learning to develop the SC character, practice answering questions in character and role-play practice in giving feedback. A follow-up personal mentoring session was also offered. These sessions provided opportunities for individual practice and to ensure that the volunteer had strategies for emotional self-protection when playing roles with many emotional and physical difficulties.

Faculty and learners

Faculty consisted of one part-time interprofessional educator (PJT) with mentors for simulation education (DN) and interprofessional practice (MB). Learners were from many different higher education institutions and included professional entry learners from medicine, nursing and allied health. Learners were selected on a convenience basis to ensure that different professions collaborated and because their placements overlapped. An administrative assistant managed bookings, data collection and the video technology for the simulations.

Preparation and briefing

Learners received pre-reading on commencement of their placement. This consisted of information on basic interprofessional competencies and a copy of the IRT. Learners usually met each other for the first time at the simulated clinic. The session was led by the interprofessional educator and initial discussion covered basic interprofessional competencies(9) and how the learners might collaborate with each other and simultaneously communicate effectively and sensitively with the SC. Discussion also covered features of client-centred interviewing and care plans. Questions on the IRT were reviewed and learners were alerted to 'red flag' points of referral and the range of health services available locally.

There were usually two simulations in each session, with two SCs booked for interview, usually an hour apart. The learners were given a limited amount of information about each client: name, sex and one or two presenting issues. Pairs of learners formed 'interprofessional teams', selected which team would interview and then planned their approach, including who would ask which questions, how they might draw on each other's strengths and practice and how they would support each other. They were given a final opportunity to ask questions about available services. Student observers were encouraged to use the IRT to structure their observations and that they would be asked to provide feedback to the learners with specific examples of behaviour.

The SCs were met by faculty and briefed on the level of learners. The SCs then changed into appropriate garments, were given an opportunity for further questions, assumed their character and took a seat in the waiting room.

The simulation

Simulations were held in the consulting rooms at two LCHS sites, in the course of the real community clinic. The SC waited with clientele in the usual waiting area until the learners entered, called their SC name and led the SC into the consulting room. The consultation was observed either though a one-way screen or via audio-visual capture. The 'interprofessional student team' introduced themselves to the SC and jointly conducted a screening interview using the IRT as a guide for questioning. By the end of the interview, learners were expected to have summarized the SC's health issues and recommended

a care plan, including referrals with respect to the client's priorities.

Debriefing and feedback

Debriefing and feedback were layered, commencing with feedback from the SC to the learners, prompted by faculty. The SCs were trained to offer structured and balanced feedback on their experiences of the learners. Once the SC feedback was completed, they left the room and the next layer of feedback was between the learner interviewers, again prompted by questions from faculty, such as:

- How did their collaboration plan go?
- What went well?
- What would they like to do differently?

The learner observers were then asked to offer feedback on the interviewing learners' interprofessional competencies. Segments of the recorded interviews were reviewed in the final layer of analysis and feedback for learners and observers. The faculty summarized the feedback with a discussion of key learning points, the objectives and what the learners might take with them into clinical practice.

Key messages

- The simulated clinics in community-based care in our rural setting provided a powerful learning opportunity for learners from different healthcare professions.
- The structured approach provided learners with safety.
- Offering the simulated clinic *in situ* provided authentic context and was highly engaging for learners, faculty and SCs.
- Basing simulated client roles on real clients added value and supported authenticity.
- Training for SCs was essential.

References

1 WHO (2010) *Framework for Action on Interprofessional Education and Collaborative Practice.* World Health Organization, Geneva.
2 Reeves S (2001) A systematic review of the effects of interprofessional education on staff involved in the care of adults with mental health problems. *Journal of Psychiatric and Mental Health Nursing,* **8**(6): 533–42.

3 Barr H (2007) Interprofessional education: the fourth focus. *Journal of Interprofessional Care*, **21**(S2): 40–50.

4 Hammick M, Freeth D, Koppel I, Reeves S and Barr H (2007) A best evidence systematic review of interprofessional education. BEME Guide No. 9. *Medical Teacher*, **29**(8): 735–51.

5 Reeves S, Zwarenstein M, Goldman J, Barr H, Freeth D, Hammick M, *et al.* (2008) Interprofessional education: effects on professional practice and health outcomes. *Cochrane Database of Systematic Reviews*, (**1**), CD002213.

6 CAIPE (2014) *Centre for Advancement of Interprofessional Education*. http://www.caipe.org.uk (accessed 7 July 2014).

7 Bridges DR, Davidson RA, Odegard PS, Maki IV and Tomkowiak J (2011) Interprofessional collaboration: three best practice models of interprofessional education. *Medical Education Online*, **16**: 6035.

8 Nestel D and Morrison T (2012) *Victorian Simulated Patient Network*. http://www.vspn.edu.au (accessed 5 November 2012).

9 Interprofessional Education Collaborative Expert Panel (2011) *Core Competencies for Interprofessional Collaborative Practice: Report of an Expert Panel*. Interprofessional Education Collaborative, Washington, DC.

16 Telephone incognito simulated patients

Jan-Joost Rethans and Hay Derkx
Maastricht University, Maastricht, The Netherlands

OVERVIEW

Many countries are now using call centres as an integral part of out-of-hours primary care. Although there has been research on safety issues within telephone consultations, there has been no published research on how to train and/or incorporate simulated patients calling for medical advice and on the accuracy of role playing. The objectives of this study were to assess the feasibility and validity of using telephone incognito simulated (standardized) patients (TISPs) and the accuracy of role plays and the rate of detection, and to explore the experiences of being a TISP and the difficulties encountered with self-recording the calls. Twelve TISPs were trained in role play by presenting their problem to a general practitioner and a nurse and to self-record calls. Calls were made to 17 different out-of-hours centres from home. Of the four or five calls per evening, one call was assessed for accuracy of role play. Retrospectively, the out-of-hours centres were asked whether they had detected any calls made by a TISP. The TISPs filled in a questionnaire concerning their training, the self-recording technique and personal experiences. The results indicated that the TISPs made 375 calls during 84 evenings and the accuracy of the role play was close to 100%. A TISP was called back the same evening for additional information in 11 cases. Self-recording caused extra tension for some TISPs. All fictitious calls remained undetected. We conclude that TISPs can be valuable for both training and assessment of performance in telephone consultation carried out by doctors, trainees and other personnel involved in medical services.

Rationale

An important part of healthcare providers' clinical tasks includes communication with patients by telephone. Communication by telephone between a patient and a healthcare professional differs from 'live' meetings or 'live consultations' with patients in the following aspects:
- There is no visual, no body and no olfactory contact between the caller (patient) and the healthcare professional (call handler).
- Physical examination is not possible.

In The Netherlands, a special type of telephone contact takes place in so-called out-of-hours (OOH) centres: patients contact these centres outside normal daytime working hours. The 'call handlers' in these centres must triage the incoming calls in terms of assessing the urgency of the problem. Depending on the healthcare context, several different options are available, including telephone-only advice or requesting that the patient visit the OOH. More than 105 OOH centres deliver primary care to a population of 17 million people. They are responsible for answering all incoming patient telephone calls. The call handlers are either a physician assistant or a nurse. We were interested in assessing the quality of telephone triage at OOH centres in The Netherlands, in order to identify any improvements to call handler training.

In general, there are *direct* and *indirect* methods of researching the healthcare delivery(1). With direct methods, the researcher can see or hear the patient–healthcare professional interaction. In indirect methods, the researcher has no direct access to these interactions and uses instead written case vignettes, surveys, interviews, etc. There is evidence that direct methods are preferred,

Simulated Patient Methodology: Theory, Evidence and Practice, First Edition. Edited by Debra Nestel and Margaret Bearman.
© 2015 John Wiley & Sons, Ltd. Published 2015 by John Wiley & Sons, Ltd.

Table 16.1 Project overview.

Aim	Assess the quality of telephone triage in order to identify improvements
Target participants	357 respondents, selected from 17 centres
Setting	Out-of-hours (OOH) clinics; SP's own home
Programme/Session length	20–30 minutes
Simulator(s)	Telephone incognito patients

in order to understand what is really occurring in actual practice(2). For our project to assess the quality of telephone triage at OOH centres, we decided to adopt a *direct* method: telephone incognito simulated patients (TISPs)(3–6).

The SP methodology offers unique opportunities for assessment of actual healthcare practice. With 'incognito' or 'unannounced' SPs, the healthcare provider is not aware that the encounter is not with a real patient. This has proved to be a valid, reliable, acceptable and feasible instrument to assess clinical performance(7). We describe: the information provided to the OOH centres, the preparation and training of the TISPs, the self-recording of the calls, the accuracy of role playing and the personal experiences of the TISPs.

Scenario examples

An overview is presented in Table 16.1.

Permission by the OOH centres

A year before we went 'live' with the TISPs, we contacted all OOH centres in The Netherlands with a written request for permission to select them for our research project. Research has shown that an interval of sufficient time between the announcement of the project and the actual visit by an SP can prevent detection(8). The OOHs that replied positively ('Yes, we may be called by a TISP') were not informed whether they were selected and once selected were not informed when they might be called.

Scenarios

We developed seven clinical scenarios to be played by the TISPs. These scenarios were developed iteratively over several drafts with feedback and comments by a number of primary-care specialists. The cases were:

1. a child aged 5 years, suffering from fever (38.6 °C) and without other symptoms;
2. an adult with fever and symptoms similar to influenza;
3. an adult with fever, also with symptoms similar to influenza but who recently had returned to The Netherlands from an African country and taking preventive anti-malaria drugs irregularly;
4. an adult with nose bleeding and no other complaints;
5. an adult with nose bleeding but also having bruises on both arms;
6. a child vomiting for an unknown reason; and
7. a child vomiting and having had a head injury a few hours before (Box 16.1).

BOX 16.1 Example scenario – child aged 5 years is vomiting

Caller is the mother: she is worried as a few weeks ago her cousin's child, also 5 years old, was admitted to a hospital when they were abroad on holiday in Turkey for vomiting and the child needed a drip. The mother wants advice on how to handle the case herself.

Opening by caller:

  'Good evening. I have a question. My son vomited a few minutes ago. I have some paracetamol. Should I give it to him?'

Answers only to be given when asked:

• Onset	3 hours ago (around 5pm) and at 6.30pm and a few minutes ago
• Behaviour of child	normal
• Frequency of vomiting	3×
• Vomited blood	no
• Diarrhoea	no
• Abdominal pain	no

• Dehydration	drank normally last few hours 1 hour ago; no pain
◦ Drinking:	
◦ Micturatio	
• Rash	no
• Fever	no
• Headache	yes, complained of a slight headache
• Earache	no
• Stiff neck	no
• Head injury	**YES**: thank you for asking me. You have reminded me that this afternoon, he fell while he was playing. He cried a lot. I also noticed a swelling at the back of his head.
• Wrong food	no
• Medical past	no
• Family	no, no one else is ill
• Self care	none

Outcome for urgency level: child should be seen by doctor within 2 hours

We made sure that for the presented signs/symptoms in the scenarios, the outcome of the required care part of the phone call was either self-care advice or a consultation by the patient at the OOH centre within the next 6 hours. None of the calls required immediate care, ambulance transport or home visits by a physician.

Each case scenario consisted of three types of information: general, case specific and local information. General information contained all fictional personal data such as address, date of birth and mobile phone number. Case-specific information was tailored to the actual medical content of the case. This included the TISP's opening sentence, how to finish the conversation and whether the TISP was anxious or worried. This information was in accordance with normal SP role scripting. We also made a list of all questions that were likely to be asked by OOH call handlers and pre-scripted the answers.

For the local information, all TISPs received a document with a geographic map of the TISPs location where they were supposed to be on the evening that they would call the OOH, and also a geographic map of the location of the OOH centre itself.

A number of experts agreed upon standards for the clinical content to assess the quality of the phone call handling in terms of medical advice. For the assessment of quality of communication by the OOHs we used the Reason (for encounter), Information (gathered), Care (advice given), Evaluation (of the encounter) (RICE) communication list(5).

All telephone calls were scheduled between 7.00pm and 10.00pm with four or maximum five calls per evening per TISP. All telephone calls were audio recorded.

Selection and training of the TISPs

We selected a group of 14 TISPs from the pool of around 80 SPs that we normally involve in training of undergraduate medical students at the medical programme of the Faculty of Health, Medicine and Life Sciences of Maastricht University. The selection was based on TISP expertise, as assessed during routine quality assurance, and on clarity of speech. We were looking for highly experienced practitioners. The TISPs were trained in pairs and each pair was trained to play one role. This provided a spare TISP if needed and diminished the risk of being detected.

A nurse and a family physician, both working at a medical call centre, trained each TISP by being in the same room with a screen between them so they could not see each other. Special attention was paid during all training sessions to speaking in a natural way and how to express non-verbal signals such as surprise, disappointment, fear or anxiety through voice intonation. The TISPs were firmly instructed to use *only* the prescribed opening phrase and the closing phrase of the telephone call, and in how to react if invited to visit the OOH centre the same evening.

The role training lasted $1\frac{1}{2}$ hours per TISP. After their training, all TISPs made a try-out call to a medical call centre that was aware it would receive a call from a TISP. This try-out was organized to boost the self-confidence of the TISPs with respect to both performance and use of recording software. A refresher training of 1 hour was provided half way through the project.

Self-recording at home

The TISPs made their calls to OOH centres spread all over the country from their own private homes. To ensure that the OOHs were unable to read the real calling-location of the TISP on their telephone screens, the TISP received special telephone equipment. This equipment could also record the telephone interactions. The training for using the recording system lasted 1 hour and was in addition to the role-play training.

Accuracy of role play

A check of the accuracy of the role play assessed the proportion of clinical features presented correctly by the TISPs during the call. The TISPs knew that we would assess their role play but were unaware which call we would assess. After all recordings were completed, we selected the third call made per evening and the assessment was carried out by two assessors on the following criteria:

- Did the TISP:
  - open the call according the instructions?
  - give the correct answers to questions asked?
  - only give information if asked for?
  - close the call according the instructions?

To explore whether the TISPs were detected by an OOH centre, we sent a letter to all centres after all calls had been made. These asked if the OOH centres realised they were being called by a TISP and, if so, when that call was made and whether the discovery was made during or after the call.

Results

Out 103 OOH centres, 98 were willing to take part in the project and we selected 17 of these, spread all over the country. Out of 357 calls that were scheduled, 18 had to be rescheduled owing to problems with self-recording by the TISPs. The TISPs needed $1\frac{1}{2}$–2 hours per evening to make their calls. Occasionally they received a return call the same evening from an OOH centre and three times, even weeks later, some TISPs were called back by the administration of an OOH centre asking for their insurance number.

Of all 357 calls made, 84 were assessed by two assessors for accuracy of role play. We found that the opening sentence was assessed as incorrect or possibly incorrect in six cases and the closing sentence was assessed as incorrect or possibly incorrect in 19 cases.

After asking all OOHs whether they had detected any TISP, we concluded that not one TISP had been detected. Interestingly, two OOH centres were very sure about being been called by a TISP when they had not been contacted!

In terms of medical quality of telephone triage at the OOH centres, our results showed that the call handlers or triage professionals asked a mean of 54% of obligatory medical items of the agreed standards. With respect to the quality of communication, as assessed by the RICE communication list, the mean overall score of the call handlers was 35%, thus leaving much room for improvement(4).

Focus group interviews with the TISPs after the data collection

In the focus groups, the TISPs stated that they were able to handle every situation met, even those for which they were not trained. They told us that this was made possible by the intensive training with a nurse and a family physician, especially when they were called back later the same evening by a physician from the OOH centre, who was following up the case by seeking more information. Helpful factors included remembering the role accurately and knowing how to use their voices. Although they could make the calls from their own homes, the special self-recording equipment had been more stressful than the telephone interview. The precise information about the location from where they were pretending to make the call had helped their performance. Five calls per evening was their maximum, as this equated to 2–$2\frac{1}{2}$ hours of focused working. The reason why sometimes the TISP did not close the consultation as prescribed was that the call handler had closed the conversation hastily.

What did we learn?

Intensive training is critical, particularly learning the role by heart and detailed preparation for projects with TISPs, All the training sessions and other logistical and practical information provided are essential to prepare the TISPs for unexpected situations. As none of the TISPs was detected, we value our preparation of the TISPs and the actual data phase collection as sufficient. Accuracy of the TISPs performance is essential in order to be able to assess the quality of actual telephone calls by the OOHs. Based on the results of these real practice performance data, we are able to advise training programmes on the areas where their call handlers can improve themselves.

Key messages

Key successes of the programme

- We showed that TISPs in a research project are reliable, valid, acceptable and feasible.
- The real practice performance data indicate that educational programmes and feedback can be better tailored to the actual needs of the healthcare provider and the patient.

Challenges with the programme

- Presenting a range of medical problems by telephone is difficult.
- We needed to determine if TISPs are a good methodology to certify call handlers.
- Recording telephone calls may not be possible in every country, owing to privacy regulations. In The Netherlands, no ethical approval is required for this type of research.

Lessons learned

- Selection of TISPs is essential.
- Training of TISPs is essential.
- In order to keep the TISPs incognito, we advise waiting a substantial amount of time between consent and data collection.

References

1 Rethans JJ, Westin S and Hays RH (1996) Methods for quality assessment in general practice. *Family Practice*, **13**: 468–76.
2 Rethans JJ, Sturmans F, Drop R, van der Vleuten C and Hobus P (1991) Does competence of general practitioners predict their performance? Comparison between examination setting and actual practice. *BMJ*, **303**: 1377–80.
3 Derkx HP, Rethans JJE, Muijtjens AM, Maiburg BH, Winkens RA, van Rooij HG, *et al.* (2008) Quality of clinical aspects of call handling at Dutch out of hours centres: cross sectional national study. *BMJ*, **337**: a1264.
4 Derkx HP, Rethans JJE, Muijtjens AM, Maiburg BH, Winkens RA, van Rooij HG, *et al.* (2009) Quality of communication during telephone triage at Dutch out-of-hours centres. *Patient Education and Counseling*, **74**: 174–8.
5 Derkx HP, Rethans JJE, Knottnerus JA and Ram P (2007) Assessing communication skills of clinical call handlers working at an out of hours centre: the development of the RICE rating scale. *British Journal of General Practice*, **57**: 383–7.
6 Derkx HP, Rethans JJE, Maiburg BH, Winkens RA and Knottnerus JA (2009) New methodology for using incognito standardised patients for telephone consultation in primary care. *Medical Education*, **43**: 82–8.
7 Rethans JJ, Gorter S, Bokken L and Morrison L (2007) Unannounced standardised patients in real practice: a systematic literature review. *Medical Education*, **41**: 537–549.
8 Maiburg BH, Rethans JJ, van Erk IM, Mathus-Vliegen LM and van Ree JW (2004) Fielding incognito standardised patients as 'known' patients in a controlled trial in general practice. *Medical Education*, **38**: 1229–35.

17 Hybrid simulated patient methodology: managing maternal deterioration

Simon JR Cooper[1,2] and Mary Anne Biro[3]

[1]Monash University, Berwick, Australia
[2]University of Brighton, Brighton, UK
[3]Monash University, Clayton, Australia

OVERVIEW

Concerns have been raised about midwives' 'failure to rescue' and their ability to manage maternal deterioration, with questions over clinical skills and knowledge and the implications for morbidity and mortality. With these issues in mind, we worked with simulated patients (SPs) to examine student midwives' ability to assess and manage maternal deterioration using measures of knowledge, skill, situation awareness and decision-making. SPs wearing 'birthing suits' simulated women in maternal deterioration. In total 35 students were assessed. Knowledge scores averaged 75% (range 46 – 91%) but skill performance was low, averaging 54% (range 39 – 70%) and with notable performance decrements as the women's condition deteriorated. Students' evaluations indicated significant benefits of the programme and the high psychological fidelity of the scenarios and SPs.

Rationale

There are significant concerns over the management of acutely deteriorating patients, with poor management of patient deterioration leading to high levels of morbidity and expensive and often unsuccessful resuscitation procedures(1,2). In midwifery, simulation has been found to improve students' decision-making and confidence(3) and, importantly, to improve medical residents' clinical performance in vaginal breech births(4).

Since 2008, using an educational model known as FIRST2ACT(5), we have run a series of exploratory studies aimed at understanding how nurses and midwives manage deteriorating conditions in simulated settings(e.g. 6,7). In our first study with student nurses, we used an advanced life support manikin to simulate deteriorating patients, identifying mediocre skill performance(8). In a video review process, participants reflected on their performance and raised process concerns. A number commented on the fidelity of the setting with comments

such as 'How unrealistic. It's hard to be friendly to a dummy' and 'I wouldn't have acted like that if it was a real person.' There is clearly some truth in these comments; manikins were originally designed for resuscitation simulation whereas we were simulating 'live' but deteriorating patients. In subsequent studies(e.g. 9), we employed SPs, with a notable reduction in concerns.

In midwifery, SPs have simulated ante-partum haemorrhage (APH) and post-partum haemorrhage (PPH) in order to gain insight into how student midwives manage acute deterioration(9). SPs were experienced professional actors who had worked in other educational simulated settings. A unique aspect of the programme was the MODEL-med birthing suit. In the APH scenarios, the SP donned a pregnancy suit with a firm uterus, while in the PPH scenarios a crying 'newborn baby' was placed beside the SP who was fitted with the MODEL-med suit (Figures 17.1 and 17.2). The suit simulates a post-partum abdomen with a palpable boggy uterus, with haemorrhage

Simulated Patient Methodology: Theory, Evidence and Practice, First Edition. Edited by Debra Nestel and Margaret Bearman.
© 2015 John Wiley & Sons, Ltd. Published 2015 by John Wiley & Sons, Ltd.

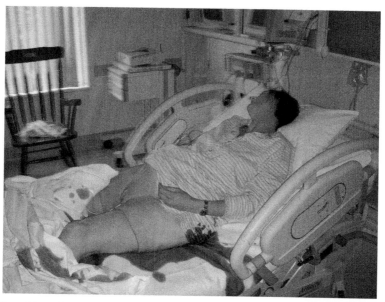

Figure 17.1 MODEL-med birthing suit.

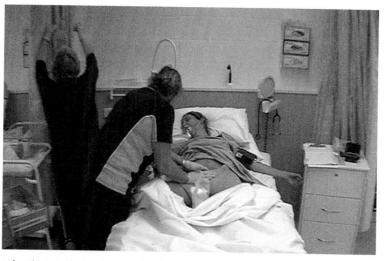

Figure 17.2 Simulated patient, student and supporting doctor.

of blood-like fluid from the vagina, and permits realistic internal examinations and procedures. Three litres of blood can be stored under the bed and using a hand-held pump the SP is able to simulate vaginal bleeding at the appropriate time. This approach significantly increased the fidelity of the scenario and enhanced learning outcomes(6).

Scenario example

The aim of this activity was to examine the ability of student midwives to assess and manage maternal deterioration using measures of knowledge, situation awareness and skill performance. Our initial objective was to assess performance and not necessarily to educate. However, it became clear from student evaluations that attendance had a significant impact on their learning. Table 17.1 presents a programme overview.

The two short scenarios (APH and PPH – incorporating the MODEL-med birthing suit) were developed from maternal records and the guidelines produced by the Royal Women's' Hospital, Melbourne. Both were then assessed by five clinical experts to ensure face and content validity. Each scenario performance was rated using an Objective Structured Clinical Examination (OSCE) template (Table 17.2), which was later used for student feedback. The objective was to understand how primary midwife first responders perform prior to the arrival of an emergency team. Scenarios therefore ran for 8 minutes. In order to mimic reality, the conduct of the simulations met two conditions:

(i) the participants were allowed to investigate freely and (ii) they were given clinical information over time but with relatively little information provided initially(10). This process-based information giving improved the ecological validity of the simulation(11) and enabled students to experience dynamic clinical thinking.

In each scenario, maternal deterioration was subtly indicated in the first 4 minutes, prior to obvious and significant deterioration in the second 4 minutes (e.g. major blood loss). In order to achieve applicable learning outcomes, two factors were taken into account: first, the predictability of relationships between variables (e.g. whether tachycardia and low blood pressure indicate hypovolaemia), and second, the level of relevant information(11). Therefore, in the PPH scenario, a

Table 17.1 Programme overview.

Overall aim	To examine the ability of student midwives to assess and manage maternal deterioration using measures of knowledge, situation awareness and skill performance
Learning objective	To enable students to reflect upon and understand their performance in an emergency setting
Target participants	Student midwives in last 6 months of study
Setting	Clinical simulation centre designed to mimic a birth suite
Program/Session length	A 2 hour session for individual participants
Faculty	Four members per session including experienced midwives, educators and researchers
Simulator	One female simulated patient of childbearing age per session (four available). All with professional acting experience and training. Actresses wore a MODEL-med birthing suit in the PPH scenario to simulate realistically the anatomy and blood loss
Frequency of offering	In this case study we describe a single offering in this format. Similar formats are now in use with simulated patients for midwifery students completing acute care study units

Table 17.2 Example of scoring from first 3 minutes of the scenario: post-partum haemorrhage.

Approximate time (minutes)	Observations	Action	Correct/ incorrect	Points at debrief
On arrival 1–3 min	Fundal check (atonic boggy uterus)		Y/N	Physiological compensation. Consider concealed blood loss
	BP 95/70	Record/request obs.	Y/N	
	HR 110		Y/N	
	RR 19		Y/N	
	CRT – 2 s		Y/N	
	O_2 sats 95%		Y/N	
		Call for help	Y/N	Consider tone, tissue, trauma, thrombin
		Identify/treat cause (*placenta and membranes delivered*)	Y/N	
				Uterus massage; ergometrine
		Massage uterus	Y/N	Prepare for IDC (*full bladder prevents uterine contractility*)
		Check blood loss (*now 1000 mL*)	Y/N	
		Give ergometrine and metoclopramide or Syntocinon	Y/N	Aware of uterine capacity to retain 1000 mL + blood/clots Ergometrine and metoclopramide or Syntocinon
		Request IDC	Y/N	

high level of relevant information was provided with a low level of uncertainty (i.e. the 'easier scenario'). In the APH scenario, less relevant information was provided and there was a higher level of uncertainty (i.e. the 'harder scenario').

Having produced the scenarios, four SPs were selected. All were professional actors in their 30s who had experienced childbirth. Prior to attending a briefing session, they were sent an outline scenario (Box 17.1), which they were able to practice with the educator and a simulated student in a 2 hour briefing. As professional actors there were few concerns over the performance, but process questions did arise, such as 'when do I do this?', 'how much pain would I be in?' and 'how should I respond to this?'

Educators were also briefed before each session (Box 17.1), but as they had assisted with the development only a brief summation was required. However, roles were allocated that required preparation. One staff member played the role of a newly qualified, inexperienced doctor who 'prescribed' or undertook medical procedures as requested. Scenario skill ratings were performed by this member of staff and a second non-participant observer. To ensure inter-rater reliability, consultation and consensus were achieved at the end of each scenario using the standardized scenario check list (Table 17.2). A third member of staff then undertook the debriefing and a fourth administered the whole session.

'Point of completion' student midwives from Monash University attended the simulation centre individually for 2 hours. The site was designed to mimic a birth suite setting. SPs acted out the two short scenarios. On arrival, each student completed a validated 11-item multiple-choice questionnaire to assess their knowledge of maternal deterioration(9). Participants were then provided with procedural information on how the scenario would run and a verbal description of the woman's presenting condition, for example 'this is a 28-year-old who has had a spontaneous vaginal birth of her first baby at term' (Box 17.1). Minimal additional information was provided initially, requiring observations and actions to be performed as the woman's condition developed. On completion of each scenario, the participant's level of situation awareness was measured using a process known as the Situation Awareness Global Assessment Technique (SAGAT)(12).

Finally, using the videoed APH and PPH scenarios, participants were debriefed using a reflective review process known as photo-elicitation(13). In this process, the participant is audio recorded whilst watching the video recordings of their performance and is 'naively' prompted by the educator with questions such as 'what were you thinking here?' and 'what did you think would happen next?'. The process reveals decision-making processes and ensures deep student reflection on their performance. Finally, an educator summarizes the 'best aspects' of performance and future 'points of improvement'. The video and audio recordings of the PPH scenario were later analysed with a focus on clinical decision-making(14).

Key messages

Outcomes
Outcomes from this programme are listed in Cooper *et al.*(9) and Scholes *et al.*(14). In summary, 35 midwifery students attended the programme. Multiple-choice knowledge test scores reached an acceptable standard overall, with an average total score of 75% (range 46–91%). However, skill performance (in the scenarios) was low. Across all items in both scenarios, participants averaged 54% (range 39–70%). Performance also decreased as the patient deteriorated, with a significant reduction in 'correct' actions in the second half of each scenario. Situation awareness scores were also low across both scenarios, averaging 54%, and in a qualitative review of the PPH scenario participants' clinical management and prioritization varied considerably.

Challenges and limitations
This was a small study of Australian midwifery students with a consequential lack of international and cultural diversity. Performance may differ in practice settings and 'simulation cannot and should not replace reality, and reality is not realised in simulation' (8, p. 2316). Participants did raise concerns about the 'unrealistic' role of the staff member who played the role of a newly qualified and inexperienced doctor, arguing that in their experience medical staff would have been more knowledgeable and proactive(14). This was a trade-off, as by reducing prompts we were able to standardize the scenarios.

BOX 17.1 Example scenario – post-partum haemorrhage

Educators/research staff

- Participants should be asked to arrive 'as for work': a uniform, notepad, pen, watch, etc., as applicable.
- Ask the participant not to discuss the scenarios with their colleagues until the study is complete.
- Ensure the demographics form is completed.
- Ensure the knowledge test is completed.
- Ensure microphone/video is correctly placed over the participant in the scenarios.
- Simplify the room and monitoring (to average birth suit setting) with BP and O_2 saturation monitoring available.
- Brief 'newly qualified doctor' (the second staff member in the scenarios) to support appropriately but without prompts, i.e. they can increase the infusion rate if requested.
- Run through the scenario with student and ask them to repeat it back.
- Explain to each participant that they will be working with an SP – they are required to take vital signs but results will be supplied by their 'medical assistant'.
- At the end of each scenario, immediately withdraw participants for situation awareness questioning.

Student

You are a newly qualified midwife who has just arrived for her shift on the birth suite. You are the only available member of qualified staff on duty (an attending midwife has just left to manage an emergency), but you have the support of a junior doctor who will assist and support as required. You are required to take observations as per normal but results will be revealed by the doctor. The woman is in a quiet side ward.

The woman

Lisa, a 28-year-old, has had a spontaneous vaginal birth of her first baby at term; the third stage has been actively managed with 10 units of intramuscular Syntocinon. She is awaiting transfer to the postnatal unit. You have been asked to do her last set of observations before transfer.

The scenario will be run in 'real time'. There will therefore be gaps in activity (this does not mean you are doing anything wrong). An observation chart is available for you to make records. Talk through what you are thinking and doing. You can ask for the woman's status at any point and you can fully expose her and perform internal vaginal examinations.

At the end of the scenario, you will be asked questions about specific aspects of the situation, as you perceive them, at that time. The questions should be answered as rapidly as possible – it is OK to use your instinct.

Patient Scenario

You are 28 years old, named Lisa, and you have just had a spontaneous vaginal birth of your first baby at term; the third stage was actively managed with 10 units of intramuscular Syntocinon. You are waiting to transfer to the postnatal unit. Your attending midwife has just left to help in an emergency. You notice that you are losing a lot of blood and express concerns to the new midwife as she arrives (release 1000 mL from pregnancy suit). You are initially alert but between minutes 4 and 7 of the scenario release an additional 800–1000 mL of blood, respond only to voice and become 'shocked' and a little disorientated. However, by the end of the scenario (7–8 minutes) you are beginning to recover, unless no applicable treatments have been performed.

Supporting doctor - role

DO NOT PROMPT at any point. Give information as requested after an applicable action, i.e. only indicate the BP or HR after the midwife has taken it. You may indicate estimated blood loss when requested. Please rate performance on the following scale (refer to Table 17.2) during or immediately after each scenario.

Ensuring consistency between scenarios can be difficult with SPs. In this study we employed one SP for each day's work, requiring rapid 'character' changes between scenarios and up to 10 scenarios per day (five students completing two scenarios each). This led to some fatigue, with possible errors and consistency issues. Employing four different SPs across the study may also have led to some inconsistency, and the interactions between the SPs and participant meant that there were some minor differences between each scenario. In summary, there is a trade-off between fidelity and replicability in this situation.

Lessons learnt

Simulated learning has an essential part to play in midwifery education, especially for complex skills that are rarely performed (e.g. obstetric emergencies). In our work to date, the core issue is the knowledge–practice divide. Simulation in 'believable' settings is essential, noting that high fidelity does not necessarily mean high technology. In this study, participant feedback indicated that SPs generated high psychological fidelity, demanding effective communication and empathic relationships, without the need for high technology. The birthing suit added to the fidelity of the situation, enabling participants to assess fundal height, uterine contractility and blood loss, an indicator which demanded rapid and decisive action (Figures 17.1 and 17.2). Through the programme we were able to build an understanding of human performance in emergency situations, and students reported significant improvements in their understanding of emergency priorities(6).

References

1 Draycott TJ, Crofts JF, Ash JP, Wilson LV, Yard E, Sibanda T, *et al.* (2008) Improving neonatal outcome through practical shoulder dystocia training. *Obstetrics and Gynecology*, **112**: 14–20.
2 Harrison GA, Jacques TC, Kilborn G and McLaws M-L (2005) The prevalence of recordings of the signs of crit-

ical conditions and emergency responses in hospital wards – the SOCCER study. *Resuscitation*, **65**: 149–57.
3 Cioffi J, Purcal N and Arundell F (2005) A pilot study to investigate the effect of a simulation strategy on the clinical decision making of midwifery students. *Journal of Nursing Education*, **44**: 131–4.
4 Deering S, Brown J, Hodor J and Satin AJ (2006) Simulation training and resident performance of singleton vaginal breech delivery. *Obstetrics and Gynaecology*, **107**: 86–9.
5 Buykx P, Kinsman L, Cooper S, McConnell-Henry T, Cant R, Endacott R, *et al.* (2011) FIRST²ACT: educating nurses to identify patient deterioration – a theory-based model for best practice simulation education. *Nurse Education Today*, **31**(7): 687–93.
6 Buykx P, Cooper S, Kinsman L, Endacott R, Scholes J, McConnell-Henry T, *et al.* (2012) Patient deterioration simulation experiences: impact on teaching and learning. *Collegian*, **19**(3): 125–9.
7 Endacott R, Scholes J, Cooper S, McConnell-Henry T, Porter J, Missen K, *et al.* (2012) Identifying patient deterioration: using simulation and reflective review to examine decision making skills in a rural hospital. *International Journal of Nursing Studies*, **49**(6): 710–7.
8 Cooper S, Kinsman L, Buykx P, McConnell-Henry T, Endacott R and Scholes J (2010) Managing the deteriorating patient in a simulated environment: nursing students' knowledge, skill, and situation awareness. *Journal of Clinical Nursing*, **19**(15): 2309–18.
9 Cooper S, Bulle B, Biro MA, Jones J, Miles M, Gilmour C, *et al.* (2012) Managing women with acute physiological deterioration: student midwives performance in a simulated setting. *Women and Birth*, **25**. 27–36.
10 Barrows H and Feltovich P (1987) The clinical reasoning process. *Medical Education*, **21**: 86–91.
11 Cioffi J (2001) Clinical simulations: development and validation. *Nurse Education Today*, **21**: 477–86.
12 SA Technologies (2014) *Super SAGAT: Situational Awareness Global Assessment Technique.* http://www.satechnologies.com (accessed 8 July 2014).
13 Harper D (1994) On the authority of the image: visual methods at the crossroads. In: Denzin N and Lincoln Y (eds) *Handbook of Qualitative Research*, pp. 403–12. Sage, Thousand Oaks, CA.
14 Scholes J, Endacott R, Biro MA, Bulle B, Cooper S, Miles M, *et al.* (2012) Clinical decision-making: midwifery students' recognition of and response to, post-partum haemorrhage in the simulation environment. *BMC Pregnancy and Childbirth*, **12**: 19.

18 Learning intimate examinations: the specialist role of Gynaecological Teaching Associates

Karen M Reynolds[1], Jim Parle[1] and Shirin Irani[2]

[1]University of Birmingham, Birmingham, UK
[2]Heart of England NHS Foundation Trust and University of Birmingham, Birmingham, UK

OVERVIEW

This is a case study of a Gynaecological Teaching Associates (GTA) teaching programme with year 3 undergraduate medical students at the University of Birmingham. It explains how the programme started, how the GTAs are recruited, what teaching the students receive, why they receive this teaching and how the students evaluate the teaching. This case study will be a useful resource for those planning on starting a GTA programme for their students.

Rationale

Intimate physical examinations can be challenging to teach and learn. An innovative approach involves a highly specialized role for simulated patients (SPs) as Gynaecological Teaching Associates (GTAs), who teach breast and pelvic examination. These SPs are typically lay women, with an interest in education and women's health. The GTAs are trained to 'use' their own bodies to teach; learners perform the examination on the GTA and receive immediate feedback and guidance from the GTA. This approach is also used for other intimate examinations such as rectal and male genitalia examination.

The focus of this case study is on the pelvic examination and describes one GTA training process and associated approach to working with students. The University of Birmingham has a large medical school with a significant SP-based programme to prepare students for clinical placements. Anecdotal evidence suggested that medical students had insufficient opportunities to conduct female pelvic examinations. The reasons for this included patients' reluctance, embarrassment or state of illness, in addition to student embarrassment. Integrating GTAs into the curriculum gave students the opportunity to conduct the examination in *simulation*, where they could make mistakes and get feedback without the additional pressures of being in a clinical situation and with a supportive teacher, and so enabled them to overcome embarrassment. Practicing with a GTA forms part of a series of staged learning activities. After learning the theory relevant to pelvic examination, students practice psychomotor skills on a task trainer. Once they have learnt the basic skills, they then progress to working with a GTA in order to integrate communication and examination skills. Finally, they have an opportunity to examine a real patient. An overview is presented in Table 18.1.

Case example

Recruitment of GTAs

GTAs are not clinicians but, as mentioned before, typically have an interest in improving women's health. We recruited through posters placed in GP practices, through email lists and through our existing role play/simulated patient team. As the programme has matured, recruitment tends to be through 'word of mouth', with our existing GTAs recruiting new ones.

Simulated Patient Methodology: Theory, Evidence and Practice, First Edition. Edited by Debra Nestel and Margaret Bearman.
© 2015 John Wiley & Sons, Ltd. Published 2015 by John Wiley & Sons, Ltd.

Table 18.1 Programme overview.

Overall aim	To teach the students what an appropriate bimanual female pelvic examination is and to allow them to practice it on a GTA and receive feedback
Learning objectives (including skills to be acquired/refined/rehearsed, etc.)	Correct technique for a bimanual female pelvic examination Appropriate language to use when consenting/explaining to the patient
Target participants (including minimum and maximum numbers)	Year 3 undergraduate medical students
Setting	In a classroom in the medical school, that has portable screens, couch and DVD-playing facilities
Programme/Session length	2 hours
Faculty (number and experience)	1 clinical lead – obstetrician and gynaecologist 1 educational lead – 5+ years experience in a GTA programme 6 GTAs – varying experience from 2 to 5+ years
Simulator(s)	One GTA and one co-facilitator (both non-clinical)
Frequency of offering	Once, in the third year of a 5 year medical degree

Training GTAs

The programme has both an educational and a clinical lead. The educational lead is physically based at the university and is able to show the GTAs the teaching environment and the location of the equipment they will need for the sessions. She teaches group facilitation, if required. The clinical lead is based at a local hospital and focuses on the clinical aspects of the programme.

Each prospective GTA is initially invited to meet the educational lead. This allows for any misunderstandings to be corrected and also an informal assessment of suitability. After this initial meeting, if the prospective GTA and the educational lead agree that the application should proceed, then a training session with the clinical lead is arranged. At this session, after further explanation as to the requirements of being a GTA, a gynaecological assessment with a pelvic examination is conducted in order to screen for any potential health issues and for suitability for student examination, from a clinical perspective. The trainee GTA is taught about her own anatomy so that she can then use that information when she is teaching. For example, the GTA will learn whether she has a retroverted or anteverted uterus. The clinical lead ensures that the GTA can tell when her cervix is being palpated as this is an important point of feedback for the students. The examination process is also demonstrated on a plastic manikin.

The next training session lasts about 2 hours. The educational lead takes the trainee GTA through the examination process from start to finish. The examination is demonstrated on the plastic model a few times and the trainee GTA is then asked to demonstrate the bimanual pelvic examination as well. At this point, the trainee GTA is given a handbook so that she can continue to learn at home. This session can be, and is, repeated until both the trainee GTA and trainer are satisfied. Most GTAs progress through training quickly, requiring between two and five training sessions in order to become familiar with the material. The next stages of training are first, to observe a GTA teaching session, and second, to teach a session, with an experienced co-facilitator.

In our programme, GTAs do not teach while they are menstruating. We ask the GTAs to make sure that they do not accept a session when they expect to be menstruating. This is, of course, not an exact science and it can, on occasion, lead to a last-minute cancellation. We know that some programmes do not follow this rule but, as our learners are third-year undergraduate medical students who have not yet carried out a bimanual pelvic examination on a female patient, we believe that this is less confronting. The feedback from our GTAs is that this is also their preferred way of teaching.

GTA teaching sessions

During a GTA teaching session, there are usually four to six year 3 undergraduate medical students present, a GTA and a co-facilitator who is another GTA or another female member of the teaching team. It is a deliberate choice not to include a clinician. The GTA is fully trained and is highly focused on the immediate purpose of the session, which is to begin to develop the skills of the female pelvic examination. If the students ask questions and the GTA is unable to answer, she will suggest that the student asks their clinical tutor at another time.

The teaching session itself is highly structured. It starts with introductions and a session overview. The group then watches a female pelvic examination on DVD, after which the GTA demonstrates the examination on the manikin. The first time she does it silently, the second time she explains what she is doing at each step and the third time the co-facilitator simulates the voice of the patient. The students are free to ask questions throughout.

Each of the students then performs the examination on the manikin and practices what to say with the co-facilitator, while being observed by their peers. Afterwards the student is asked how they felt it went and if there is anything they would do differently. The GTA then gives the student feedback on the examination and the co-facilitator gives feedback on the communication element. The other students are then invited to give feedback to their peer.

Once all of the students have practiced on the manikin, there is usually a 10 minute break. The room is set up for the clinical examination and the GTA empties her bladder.

In the clinical examination component of the session, each student examines the GTA, while being observed by their peers. The GTA gives the student assistance and feedback throughout. The GTA will ask the student to palpate her cervix and provides guidance to assist identification. The students are also asked to identify the fundus of the uterus when palpating the abdomen during the bimanual examination. This is sometimes difficult for the students but once again the GTAs guide them. The students are often very excited once they have palpated the uterus and fundus of the uterus for the first time.

Once the examination is completed, the GTA and the other students give feedback. For almost all students this is their first time performing a bimanual female pelvic examination on a real person, so they are usually quite relieved once the examination is over.

The session ends by answering any questions and with a brief evaluation.

Evaluation

The evaluation comprises two parts. The first is based on The Gynaecologic Examination Distress Questionnaire (GyExDQ)(1). This is a questionnaire covering comfort levels before and after the examination. The examination is broken down into five distinct elements; students rate how comfortable or uncomfortable they felt performing each element before and after the session. Students are asked about palpating the abdomen and, at their level, we would expect the majority to be comfortable or very comfortable with this element. They tend to be more uncomfortable prior to the session with respect to inspecting the external female genitalia, separating the labia majora and inserting two fingers into the vagina and talking to patients while performing an intimate examination. After the session, they almost all report being 'comfortable' or 'very comfortable' with these elements.

The second part asks the students to evaluate the GTA as a teacher. Over the last few years, we have been analysing the data collected from the evaluations and we have seen some trends. Almost all of the students find the teaching session very useful and value the opportunity. Contrary to what one might expect, male and female students are equally uncomfortable with the examination before the session. Over the last couple of years the students have appeared less uncomfortable at the start of the session compared with the earlier years; we believe that this might be due to the fact that the programme is now embedded into the curriculum and is a session which is accepted and anticipated by the students.

Key messages

Key successes of the session/programme

- Each student gets a session learning how to do a bimanual female pelvic examination in a safe, supported environment. As a team, we feel it is extremely important that students learn in this way, in order to normalize gynaecological and other intimate examinations. This session helps to show them how they can overcome their embarrassment and how to perform an appropriate bimanual examination.
- The students are told that there is not a script they can learn but that they are learning to feel comfortable with the provision of information and framing questions to the patient. The students get to practice this during the session.
- Each student gets one-on-one immediate feedback.

- The students value the session, especially working with the GTAs.
- The GTAs value their work.

Challenges with the session/programme
- Recruitment of GTAs.
- Acceptance of the programme by other colleagues.
- Scheduling GTAs around their menstrual cycles.
- The students only get to examine 'normal' women with cervix and uterus intact.

Lessons learnt
- Assume there will be difficulty recruiting GTAs initially. This is very difficult to overcome and at the start it might seem insurmountable. The most important thing we found was talking about the programme whenever a suitable opportunity came up. We found that women who were interested in education and women's health were the type of women who wanted to be involved.
- Know who to recruit: for our programme, we needed women who have a cervix and a uterus, so this is part of the first conversation. It is also important to screen out women who have an underlying agenda – such as 'hammering home' a specific message to students – this will usually show up during the teaching sessions.
- Make sure there is suitable teaching space available.
- Ensure that the budget has contingency funds for extra sessions and consumables.

Reference

1 Siwe K, Klaas W, Martin S and Barbro W (2007) Medical students learning the pelvic examination: comparison of outcome in terms of skills between a professional patient and a clinical patient model. *Patient Education and Counselling*, **68**: 211–7.

19 Advanced nursing practice in aged care: developing communication and management skills in patients with Alzheimer's disease

Jennifer H Fisher[1], Jane H Kass-Wolff[2], Ernestine Kotthoff-Burrell[2] and Jeanie M Youngwerth[1]

[1]University of Colorado School of Medicine, Aurora, USA
[2]College of Nursing at the University of Colorado Anshutz Medical Campus, Aurora, USA

OVERVIEW

This case study describes a scenario developed to support advanced practice nurses managing patients with Alzheimer's disease. The scenario is centred on an ageing couple, John and Margo Atkins, and uses time compressed intervals to support nurses in their care of patients and their families.

Rationale

Our College of Nursing faculty was seeking innovative ways to enhance the geriatric nursing curriculum for advanced practice nurse learners. After receiving funding, the faculty approached the campus Simulation Center to explore experiential educational opportunities that focused on communication skills and geriatric nursing. A simulated patient (SP) scenario was developed, which begins at one point in time and extends well beyond the initial visit to include progression of Alzheimer's disease. The case of *John and Margo Atkins* meets the goals of exposing learners to *breaking bad news* and facilitating family medical decision-making. An overview is presented in Table 19.1.

Case example

The first session requires learners to break the news of the Alzheimer's diagnosis to Mrs. Margo Atkins. This is challenging for all healthcare professionals and nurses in advanced practice training are likely to be inexperienced in this skill. The second session takes place 7 years later and allows Mr. John Atkins and his son to discuss Mrs. Atkins' wishes for end-of-life care. The focus of the second session is on helping the family cope with changes in Mrs. Atkins' health status, including plans for care and dying.

Preparation
Simulation Center staff and nursing faculty met to identify goals and learning objectives and to develop the scenario. Once learner numbers had been determined and dates scheduled in the Simulation Center, the appropriate number of SPs were recruited and a training day was scheduled.

Prior to training, SPs were provided with scenario materials (Box 19.1). At the training day, critical details were reviewed and then SPs were paired and portrayals were practiced under the supervision of an SP practitioner. SPs received feedback on levels of emotion during the portrayals to ensure that the SPs would perform in a similar way. Training for the portrayal of the second session is a more challenging endeavour because of the conflict between father and adult child over Margo's future care. The SP practitioner closely monitored the SP pairs for appropriate intensity and anger levels. The final aspect of training focused on the structure of the debriefing.

Simulated Patient Methodology: Theory, Evidence and Practice, First Edition. Edited by Debra Nestel and Margaret Bearman.
© 2015 John Wiley & Sons, Ltd. Published 2015 by John Wiley & Sons, Ltd.

Table 19.1 Programme overview.

Overall aim	Provide a similar educational experience for advanced practice nursing learners to enhance skills in working with geriatric patients and their families
Learning objectives	• Enhance skill set in *delivering difficult news* to a patient with Alzheimer's or other chronic/terminal disease
	• Enhance skill set in providing supportive communication for clients and family members
	• Enhance skill set in facilitating a family meeting
	• Identify areas of strength as well as areas to improve in communication and management of patients with Alzheimer's disease
Target participants	• Advanced practice nursing learners (or medical students)
	• Minimum number of learners is 2
	• Maximum number of learners is 24
Setting	Ambulatory clinic setting within the campus Simulation Center
Program/Session length	30 minutes of preparation time for SPs
	Briefing – 15 minutes
	SP encounter – 20 minutes
	Reflection on computer – 5 minutes
	Debriefing with SPs – 10 minutes
	Debriefing with faculty – 20 minutes
Faculty	College of Nursing faculty and Palliative Care faculty with several years' clinical and instructional experience
Simulator	SPs
Frequency of offering	Annually

Feedback goals were for SPs to be learner centred, specific and focused on observable behaviours. SPs were given opportunities to practice feedback to *learners* with input and refinement from the SP practitioner.

Briefing faculty and learners

Prior to the session, learners were assigned an article on sharing difficult news that discussed a simple mnemonic ABCDE for *difficult news* discussions – **A**dvanced preparation, **B**uild a therapeutic environment/relationship, **C**ommunicate well, **D**eal with the patient and family reactions and **E**ncourage and validate emotions(1). Learners were also provided with access to information on the Five Wishes Form(2) and a paper on last wishes of patients. Learners were briefed as a group by faculty just prior to the session.

Activity logistics

This is a two-day activity that was spaced a few weeks apart. Learners were paired, with some trios due to logistical constraints. After verbal briefing with faculty, learners were given a brief orientation by Simulation Center staff on listening for the overhead timing announcements, thoroughly reading the door signs and how to use the computers for the post-encounter exercise. Learners were also instructed to designate a lead interviewer and the second team member was encouraged to add to the patient encounter as appropriate. While the SP pairs completed rating forms on the learners in encounters, each learner group was asked to complete a short reflection on the computer. The group self-assessed on the same questions that the SP pair completed on the learner group. The group then returned to the room for a debriefing with the SP pair to discuss communication skills and then met with faculty for a more in-depth discussion on content.

Debriefing

On each session day, after completing the computer rating forms, learners had the opportunity for debriefing with their SPs. The debriefing was learner centred and allowed the learner team to reflect immediately on their performance and seek input on how to enhance their communication in the future. For learners who struggled, SPs allowed the opportunity for practicing alternative approaches to the encounter.

For the faculty debriefing of learners, participants were asked to reflect on how they felt the interview with the SPs went. Specifically, the

---

BOX 19.1 Information provided to learners

Session 1

You are an Advanced Nursing Practice student working with a preceptor in clinic. Today you will be seeing a patient who is returning for an opinion regarding the cause of her cognitive difficulties. At a previous visit the patient (and her spouse) related noticing slowly progressive problems with her memory over the past year. She had a recent episode where she could not remember where her car was parked or what it looked like, which increased her concerns. She scored 26/30 on an MMSE test and early Alzheimer's disease was suspected. You and your preceptor referred the patient to a neurologist for her opinion 1 month ago. The neurologist's evaluation included laboratory work and a head MRI scan that were unremarkable, and her consultation note (sent to you; the patient does not know the results yet) agreed that the patient appears to have early Alzheimer's disease. The patient and her spouse return today to be informed about your opinion/conclusion regarding her diagnosis and to begin to address questions, concerns, care plans, etc.

Note: You should not focus on taking an extensive history and you should not perform a physical examination.

The goal of today's visit is to inform the patient of her diagnosis and prognosis in a supportive, empathetic and relationship-centred way.

Session 2

You are now an Advanced Nursing Practice faculty member. John and Margo transferred their care to you after your former preceptor retired and they continue to be your patients. Margo now has severe dementia. She rarely speaks and frequently does not recognize her family. She has had several hospitalizations recently and is currently in hospital with aspiration pneumonia. Since admission, she is unable to control her own secretions and is not able to eat or drink without aspiration. She has pulled out multiple tubes and IVs. She has severe agitation and is requiring either sedatives or restraints to continue to provide her with the current level of care. Treatment for pneumonia shows no improvement and she is hypoxic. New complications are emerging – worsening kidney function, electrolyte abnormalities and delirium. Although currently not requiring support, you would not be surprised if she died within a fortnight. The inpatient team would like to clarify her goals of care. The inpatient medical team has been discussing end-of-life issues with John and his child. The medical team is feeling frustrated because the family cannot agree on a management plan. John feels that they should move towards comfort measures. *John and Margo's child would like aggressive interventions including intubation.* The inpatient team and John have both requested a family meeting.

You will be meeting with John and his son. The goal of the visit is to help them move toward consensus. You do not need to make any specific decisions today. You just need to begin the conversation – elicit their concerns, focus on the patient's goals of care and explore areas of family alignment.

---

group was asked what went well, what did not go as well and areas they thought they could improve. The purpose of the group debrief was to allow the learners the opportunity to learn from others and to be able to seek clinical content *pearls* from the faculty. Faculty was also able to provide anecdotes and stories to reinforce the learning objectives and answer questions.

Key messages

Successes

- College of Nursing perspective – The Advanced Practice Nursing learners have little prior experience of working with SPs and most thought this was an excellent way to learn. The activity was not assessed and therefore was less

threatening to learners. The learners and faculty saw it as a means of rehearsing before real clinical practice. Learners thought the group debriefing was helpful because hearing what others thought they did well or not so well helped each learner understand that these interactions are difficult and there is no one right way.
- Simulation Center perspective – Engagement with a new user group.

Challenges
- College of Nursing perspective – It was challenging for the faculty to add a curricular activity into a pre-existing course. There was also time spent on scheduling and informing learners about the timing of the new activity. Learners expressed a desire to have more discussion prior to the SP-based scenario about the process of doing this type of educational activity. Simulation on the campus is charged by event and is not subsidized. Faculty felt pressure from their leadership to justify the cost of the educational activity.
- Simulation Center perspective – The course faculty had asked for reports on the learner teams, but due to electronically based scheduling and late changes the data were compromised. Scheduling logistics meant significant downtime for SPs, resulting in higher costs of the programme.

Lessons learned
- College of Nursing perspective – Nursing faculty would like to increase SP-based activities to develop key concepts in communication, clinical reasoning and patient assessment. Increase the nursing faculty debriefing time.
- Simulation Center perspective – New users of simulation modalities often have anxiety; this was manifested through many questions during the briefing. Ensure sufficient time is allocated.

References

1 VandeKieft G (2001) Breaking bad news. *American Family Physician*, **64**(15): 1975–8.
2 Aging with Dignity (2013) *Five Wishes*. http://www.agingwithdignity.org/legal_Colorado.php (accessed 14 April 2014).

20 Skills development in person-centred physiotherapy

Felicity C Blackstock[1] and Shane Pritchard[2]

[1]La Trobe University, Bundoora, Australia
[2]Monash University, Clayton, Australia

OVERVIEW

Simulating the role of a patient is not new to physiotherapy education, with students having practiced skills on each other for many years. However, there have been limitations with this learning experience and entry-level physiotherapy education is now incorporating simulated patients (SPs). Internationally, SPs have contributed to the training of physiotherapists and this has increased in recent years with the development of new technologies and educational design. This chapter describes an exemplar curriculum with SPs in the development of person-centred practice for physiotherapy students during their preclinical learning.

Rationale

Simulating the role of a patient is not new to physiotherapy education: physiotherapy students have been 'patients' for their peers for many years, prior to entering the clinical environment. This role play has some disadvantages: there is often little realism; roles are usually not age matched, student patients are still learning about the movement disorder they are intending to portray; and the familiarity of peers often distracts students.

Chapter 2 detailed the diverse scope of practice of Sps. This can be translated to physiotherapy education, with patient roles developed to facilitate skill development in professional behaviour, effective communication, patient assessment, clinical reasoning and analysis, and performing and evaluating an intervention. SPs communicate and portray movement disorders with a degree of realism and authenticity that is not possible with other simulation and role-play modalities.

Published literature on the contribution of SPs to physiotherapy education is sparse. However, the available literature describes SP programme uptake in many domains of physiotherapy practice: musculoskeletal, neurological and cardiorespiratory fields, in acute, sub-acute and chronic patient populations[1–6]. Most papers have reported the use of a study-designed post-programme survey to evaluate the experience. Physiotherapy students enjoy interacting with SPs and consistently feel more confident and less anxious[1,3–6]. The literature does not demonstrate whether incorporating an SP programme is more effective than other educational methods. However, two recent randomized controlled trials demonstrated that SP interactions can replace traditional clinical placement learning time by up to 25%, with a comparable attainment of competency to practice[5,6]. The students who completed the SP activities also reported the experience to be very positive. It is clear that the theory and evidence for incorporating SPs into physiotherapy education are growing.

Surveys of entry-level physiotherapy programmes in the United States and Canada[7] and in Australia[8] have found that SP programmes embedded in curricula are increasing. However, both reported that excessive cost and a lack of availability of resources and training were significant barriers.

In this chapter, we detail an innovative, cost-effective SP programme embedded in an

Simulated Patient Methodology: Theory, Evidence and Practice, First Edition. Edited by Debra Nestel and Margaret Bearman.
© 2015 John Wiley & Sons, Ltd. Published 2015 by John Wiley & Sons, Ltd.

Table 20.1 Programme overview.

Overall aim	The subject and SP interactions aim to facilitate students' professional practice skills, including the development of communication and rapport with patients, person-centred clinical decision-making and ethical, professional and safe practice in a supportive experiential learning environment
Learning objectives	At the end of the subject, student will be able to:
	• Apply effective communication skills for the purpose of gaining informed consent, engaging a person in a therapeutic alliance for person-centred clinical assessment and interventions and recording these procedures to satisfy medico-legal requirements
	• Apply person-centred clinical reasoning skills, with reference to professional conduct, ethics and safety, to identify relevant and detailed information and develop person-centred treatment strategies, from a range of clinical scenarios
	• Perform a case-sensitive analysis and interpretation of clinical assessment findings relevant to a range of clinical scenarios, to produce a person-centred prioritized problem list
	• Formulate a discharge plan that has drawn on the therapeutic alliance and facilitates self-management as appropriate, for a range of clinical scenarios
	• Demonstrate different writing skills for different contexts and audiences within the healthcare setting
Target participants	Third- year (of 4 years) undergraduate physiotherapy students and first-year (of 2 years) graduate entry Master of Physiotherapy Practice students completing preclinical curriculum
Setting	Simulated acute hospital ward, physiotherapy inpatient rehabilitation gymnasium and physiotherapy outpatient department
Programme	• Four 2 hour sessions with the simulated patient and accompanying workshop-based learning, simulation scenario orientation/briefing and debriefing sessions, totalling 39 hours of face-to-face learning
	• In the first session, students meet their patient and conduct a patient interview. The second session focuses on motivational interviewing. In the third session, students conduct a risk assessment to determine the most appropriate methods for assisting their patient from A to B (for example, from bed to chair), minimizing the risk of harm and fostering a safe work culture. In the final session, students complete a full assessment (patient interview and appropriate outcome measures), develop a prioritized problem list and treatment plan and implement their treatment plan with the SP. The underpinning focus of all sessions is person-centred care. Debriefing includes feedback from the actors, viewing of videos of the simulated patient interaction and use of structured reflection and assessment tools
Faculty	• A total of three faculty staff across two campuses of delivery
	• Within each simulation, 20 students are involved and grouped together to be approximately five with a 'patient'. One faculty staff supervisors the interaction and facilitates the debriefing
Simulator(s)	Simulated patients
Frequency of offering	• The subject is offered annually to all entry-level physiotherapy students (totalling 150 per annum)
	• Class number is 20. Total of 8 classes for cohort of physiotherapy students per annum

entry-level physiotherapy curriculum. Table 20.1 presents an overview.

Case example

Skills development for person-centred physiotherapy

A 39 hour face-to-face preclinical subject, *Skills Development for Person-Centred Physiotherapy*, was designed and implemented in 2011. The subject is underpinned by the principles of enquiry-based learning, where students are encouraged to learn through experience, ask questions and think holistically. The subject incorporates a fictional hospital and patient caseload, where students are junior physiotherapists responsible for the care of a specific patient. Students are allocated to one of four different patient scenarios integrated into the learning activities and work within a team of five peers discussing directions of patient care. Students interact with their SP on four separate occasions during the 12 week university semester. Details are given in Box 20.1.

BOX 20.1 Example scenario: pelvic fracture

Maybelle Cheng, a 77-year-old woman, was involved in a high-speed car accident just outside Mildura in regional Victoria. She was driving to visit her only daughter (only child from a previous marriage, her first husband died 15 years ago from a heart attack) and her family who live in Mildura. Maybelle's husband (Paul Xiu Wen Cheng) was driving and it was dusk when a kangaroo jumped onto the road in front of the vehicle. Paul swerved to avoid the animal, but lost control of the vehicle and it hit a tree. Assistance was immediate from a passing car, but Maybelle was trapped in the car for 20 minutes before the rescue team were able to free her. She sustained a fracture of the pelvis and minor lacerations to her left arm and leg. Paul was critically injured, with multiple fractures and internal bleeding. Both Maybelle and Paul were flown from Mildura to Melbourne and admitted to the trauma centre. The doctors were able to attend to Maybelle's lacerations with just dressings and the pelvic fracture has been managed conservatively with bed rest (Maybelle is non-weight bearing for 6 weeks – meaning she must remain in bed or a wheel chair all day, every day for this time period). Paul required major surgery and intensive care unit management. It is now 2 weeks since the accident and Maybelle has been transferred to a private rehabilitation hospital. The costs of healthcare needs are being met by TAC – the Transport Accident Commission. Paul remains in intensive care at the acute hospital and is still very unwell. Maybelle is unsure whether her beloved husband of 10 years is going to survive.

Maybelle's character:

- When you were first admitted the pain in your pelvis was very intense, you were unable to sleep without heavy pain medication and every movement caused you pain.
- Now your pain is only present when you try to move your legs or sit up in bed.
- You are dependent on the nurses assisting you with most things – showering on a commode chair, moving out of bed into a wheel chair, dressing.
- You are not able to walk at all – the nurses use a hoist to get you out of bed into a chair. You cannot sit for long in a chair as you begin to have pain after about 20 minutes and find it uncomfortable.

- You can move your arms the full amount, but your legs only move about 50% of their full range.
- You slowly feel you are getting weaker as you haven't been doing anything. Your legs and arms are feeling heavy to lift. You fatigue easily when trying to get dressed.
- You are normally a reasonably active person, you live in Melbourne with Paul in a retirement village villa. Normally you are able to cook, clean, shop (albeit slowly) and look after yourself and Paul without any problems.
- Emotionally you are low – Paul is still very unwell, you feel alone as your family is in Mildura and you don't like being dependent on others for assistance. Friends do visit, but you miss Paul, you haven't seen him in a few days (the nurses would take you to the ICU to sit by his bed) and won't be able to now that you are in another hospital. You are easily distracted because of this.
- You also have a slight hearing difficulty, you need to tell anyone who speaks softly to talk up. You also find it difficult to remember the little things.
- You have no other significant medical issues and this is your first significant hospital admission.

The SP is a professional actor, selected from an SP database specifically for the role based on their age, gender and physical attributes. SPs are provided with a detailed description of the role 1 month prior to the first session. A 2 hour training session is conducted 2 weeks prior to the first session to calibrate the role among SPs and to provide training for SPs in providing feedback.

The greatest challenge is the development of physical attributes. To facilitate the development of movement dysfunction, faculty demonstrate the movement, videos of patients with the specific characteristics are viewed and, if possible and appropriate, people with the condition to be portrayed attend the training session. Faculty provide extensive feedback during rehearsal. SPs are trained to give feedback on their experience as a patient, not specific physiotherapy skills.

SPs attend a 30 minute briefing on the day of the simulation while students complete an online orientation to the SP interaction by downloading a video capture. The video includes a demonstration of faculty staff with an SP, shows the students the simulated environment and illustrates the use of the time in/time out procedure.

During the simulation, the five students interact with the SP simultaneously to encourage peer support and learning. Faculty supervise the interaction and participate in time out discussions, providing feedback to students on performance and guiding the development of clinical decision-making skills. The debrief process is conducted in two parts. Immediately following the simulation, the SP comes out of character and provides feedback to the students as a group for sessions 1, 3 and 4. In session 2, the SP provides individual feedback to each student. The SP also allocates a mark out of 10 for performance in communication and professionalism, which contributes to the student's official academic grade. Therefore, students receive formal feedback on their capability to develop a person-centred approach to clinical practice from the 'patient' themselves.

The second component of the debrief is conducted in their small groups during a 1 hour tutorial held the week following the simulation. Students are video recorded during the interaction with their 'patient' and the students then view the video. The same faculty staff member who facilitated the simulation facilitates this session. Students reflect on their performance using the assessment criteria that future clinical educators will apply when the student progresses to the clinical learning environment(9). This has the benefit of students developing reflective practice skills and insight into their performance and also being orientated to their future assessment criteria for physiotherapy clinical practice in the following semesters.

Separate from the debrief sessions, feedback is given to the actors on their performance and student feedback skills by faculty staff who facilitated the SP interaction.

The subject *Skill Development for Person-Centred Physiotherapy* has been extremely well received by students, with specific feedback from them about the rich experience of working with SPs and having assessment directly related to their development of skills relevant to future practice as a physiotherapist. The students have rated the overall quality of the subject over the 3 years as between 4.1 and 4.6 out of 5. Evaluation data indicate that the learning experience is supportive yet engaging and that it gives students the opportunity to prepare themselves for continuing on into the clinical practice environment.

Key messages

The challenges specific to working with SPs in physiotherapy education are around the realism of the scenario being played by the 'patient' (actor, volunteer or physiotherapy student). Physiotherapy practice relies heavily on observation of movement and dysfunction identification. Should movement and any associated pain experience not be accurately portrayed by the 'patient', the scenario can take a significantly different track and the learners can become confused. Training and rehearsal are paramount to accurate portrayal and a learning experience that aligns with the learning objectives.

Integrating SP interactions into the preclinical physiotherapy curriculum enables students a safe learning opportunity to speak to a 'patient', assess a 'patient' and treat a 'patient' before they interact with a real patient on clinical placement. This case study describes an innovative, cost-effective approach demonstrating that SPs can be successfully embedded into entry-level physiotherapy education.

Tips for successful implementation in physiotherapy

- Videos of real patients with the movement disorder or pain provide the SP with context.
- Props such a hat or scarf can be very helpful for the SP to get 'in role.' Consider restraining movement through the use of orthoses/bandages/strapping tape, e.g. collar and cuff for shoulder hemiplegia.
- Practice is paramount for the SP. Provide lots of feedback to the SP on how to display the desired attributes and interpret pain on movement.
- Encouraging the SPs to remember a time when they had pain can help with calibration of reaction.

References

1 Black B and Marcoux BC (2002) Feasibility of using standardized patients in a physical therapist education program: a pilot study. *Journal of Physical Therapy Education*, **16**: 49–56.

2 Cahalin LP, Markowski A, Hickey M and Hayward L (2011) A cardiopulmonary instructor's perspective on a standardized patient experience: implications for cardiopulmonary physical therapy education. *Cardiopulmonary Physical Therapy Journal*, **22**: 21–30.

3 Lewis M, Bell J and Asghar A (2008) Use of simulated patients in development of physiotherapy students' interpersonal skills. *International Journal of Therapy and Rehabilitation*, **15**: 221–7.

4 Wamsley M, Staves J, Kroon L, Topp K, Hossaini M, Newlin B, *et al.* (2012) The impact of an interprofessional standardized patient exercise on attitudes toward working in interprofessional teams. *Journal of Interprofessional Care*, **26**: 28–35.

5 Watson, K, Wright A, Morris N, McMeeken J, Rivett D, Blackstock F, *et al.* (2012) Can simulation replace part of clinical time? Two parallel randomised controlled trials. *Medical Education*, **46**: 657–67.

6 Blackstock FC, Watson KM, Morris NR, Jones A, Wright A, McMeeken JM, *et al.* (2013) Simulation can contribute a part of a cardiorespiratory physiotherapy clinical education: two randomized trials. *Simulation in Healthcare*, **8**: 32–42.

7 Paparella-Pitzel S, Edmond S and DeCaro C (2009) The use of standardized patients in physical therapist education programs. *Journal of Physical Therapy Education*, **23**: 15–23.

8 Jull G, Wright A, McMeeken J, Morris N, Rivett D, Blackstock F, *et al.* (2010) *National Simulated Learning Project Report for Physiotherapy*. Health Workforce Australia.

9 Dalton M, Davidson M and Keating J (2011) The Assessment of Physiotherapy Practice (APP) is a valid measure of professional competence of physiotherapy students: a cross-sectional study with Rasch analysis. *Journal of Physiotherapy*, **57**: 239–46.

21 Simulated family and healthcare professionals: consent for organ transplantation

Gayle A Gliva-McConvey

Eastern Virginia Medical School, Norfolk, USA

OVERVIEW

This chapter describes how simulated patient (SP) methodology can be used to train personnel who work with potential organ donor families. A curriculum integrating the knowledge of organ donation processes and the application of communication techniques, including assessment and feedback, using SP activities was developed. The materials illustrate how SP methodology can support complex communication skills in a highly emotional topic area.

Rationale

A national USA Organ Procurement Organization, which coordinates the recovery and transplant of organs, wanted to offer a comprehensive training programme for their new patient advocates or Family Support Coordinators (FSCs). The role of the FSC is to navigate through the total process with a positive outcome of organ donation: from the death of a person, discussions with physicians and nurses and finally approaching the donor family. In Virginia, if a person has not already registered their decision regarding organ donation on a state register, the legal next of kin (NOK) is responsible for the organ donation decision. Therefore, it is critical to establish effective strategies and skills to work with potential donors and healthcare professionals. A foundation of the programme was the balance between establishing an emotional connection with the family and strengthening the professional relationships with the physician and nurses. The SP methodology was ideal for this training owing to the highly emotional and sensitive nature of the encounters and the impact of the desired outcomes (informed consent). The training programme was designed to use the SP methodology to train the FSC to work with simulated next of kin, simulated physicians and simulated nurses. This allowed the FSC to gain experience with the total process prior to working in a real environment.

During the educational activity, the FSC practiced those aspects of the core concepts and guidelines needed for important communication skills. The programme focused on the skills relevant to obtaining consent from family members for organ and tissue transplantation in addition to skills for working with challenging healthcare providers. These included the development of rapport and relationships, ability to educate family members and health professionals, health promotion and partnership, time management and working with diverse populations. A programme overview is presented in Table 21.1.

Case example

Educational activity

The Course Planner collaborated with the Organ Procurement Organization's training team in Virginia to design a comprehensive educational activity that integrated both large group lectures and individual simulated interactions with immediate feedback. The training team produced long- and

Simulated Patient Methodology: Theory, Evidence and Practice, First Edition. Edited by Debra Nestel and Margaret Bearman.
© 2015 John Wiley & Sons, Ltd. Published 2015 by John Wiley & Sons, Ltd.

Table 21.1 Programme overview.

Overall aims	To improve consent outcomes while respecting the next of kin and their period of bereavement and to develop professional relationships with healthcare providers.
Learning objectives	On completion of the simulation, the FSC will be able to
	• define the relationships of the FSC (patient advocate) with families and health providers;
	• identify the core concepts of partnering with a health provider and families and apply strategies to strengthen the professional relationships when working with challenging personalities;
	• demonstrate skills and confidence when establishing a professional and emotional connection with the family
Target participants	Novice Family Support Coordinators
Setting	Intensive Care Unit
Programme/Session length	6 hours
Faculty	Two trainers, SPs
Simulator(s)	Simulated family and simulated healthcare professionals
Frequency of offering	Biannually

short-form didactic materials that covered a range of topics, including:

• Preparation and interaction with healthcare providers (HCPs);
• being sensitive to the family;
• verbal and non-verbal communication techniques;
• managing yourself in a crisis; and
• finding your own words for expressing empathy.

All topics were implemented into checklists for the SPs to use in assessing the FSC and reinforced in the simulated activities. Box 21.1 gives a sample scenario and Table 21.2 lists sample checklist items.

There were four to six simulation sessions, each lasting for 45 minutes. The sessions comprised:

• 10 minutes of interaction with the HCP;
• 20 minutes of interaction with next of kin;
• 20 minutes of individualized feedback/debriefing.

Assessment

The simulated family and simulated healthcare professionals completed checklists and comments to be used during the debriefing phase. Individual educational reports, which were prepared by the SP Educator, were sent to the participants after the activity. The FSCs were required to view their own performances after the educational activity for self-assessment and to provide comments. Their personal assessment and comments were reviewed by the organization's manager.

The FSCs completed a survey before and after the sessions, which were used to modify and refine activities.

Success of the activity

It is difficult to assess the success of educational activities that are based on the development of communication skills and how they influence performance in the daily practices of the learner. However, there was a significant increase in the consent rates for donation by real families after each of the educational activities conducted using simulation. This trend was documented over a 3 year period and continues to provide support for the success of the training.

The feedback from the FSCs was very positive and they felt that the experience would easily be transferred into real situations.

The FSCs appreciated the opportunity to practice the 'educational' component when preparing for and interacting with healthcare providers. Several FSCs tried multiple approaches during the activity to explore techniques and approaches that worked for them. Confidence ratings by the FSCs increased pre- and post-activity.

Key messages

Challenges and lessons learnt

The selection of the SPs for any role is critical to the success of the activity. The demographics for age, gender, ability to work as a realistic family and within the family dynamics and portray highly emotional roles are always essential for

BOX 21.1 Sample scenario: request to wait for brain death

Setting

Intensive Care Unit – daughter of the patient is in the waiting room with her husband. The daughter is very tearful, with husband being supportive of her.

Opening Statement

(Daughter's response to FSC query) 'I just can't believe this is happening, dad and I were doing our morning run to train for the upcoming marathon and he just grabbed his head and screamed out, then fell to the ground.' He was feeling great this morning, had no complaints and was laughing and talking the whole time we were running.'

Relevant information

Neurosurgeon has spoken with the daughter and her husband regarding her father's condition. He explained the ruptured aneurysm with massive bleeding into the brain, as well as the bleed being inoperable. The daughter and her husband have been in to see her father and were surprised that he looked like he's just sleeping. The patient is not yet brain dead; he occasionally breathes over the vent. He is not on the Donate Life Virginia Registry.

History of donor's condition

Patient was running with his daughter this morning around 8.00am, training for their upcoming marathon. He had been running for 30 minutes with no complaints and had been talking prior to grabbing his head and screaming out. He immediately fell to the ground and lost consciousness as his daughter was trying to support him. The driver of a passing car stopped and called 911. EMS arrived, stabilized him and transported him to the local hospital. Upon arrival he was intubated/placed on a ventilator; head

CT showed a ruptured aneurysm with mass effect. Neurosurgeon was consulted and determined the ruptured aneurysm and bleeding were inoperable.

History of physician–family relationship

The neurosurgeon has given grave prognosis and the option to withdraw support. He explained that the patient would probably be brain dead with 24 hours. The physician was giving the family some time and has not ordered any medications to support the patient's blood pressure since this would be futile. Family did decide to make him a DNR. The daughter and her husband understand the prognosis and are considering their option to withdraw support.

Next of kin (NOK) presentation/affect

NOK is very tearful and emotional at times. She wonders if she could have known/could have done something. Also, she was the one who suggested that they train for and participate in the marathon – and is feeling some guilt for that. Son-in-law is basically calling the shots by asking his wife questions and prompting and/or assuming the answers. Often during a family meeting, she sits and cries with her head down – seeming not to listen, and he presents proposed actions/re-verbalizes what was said/asks if she understand, and she often simply nods or shakes her head. Son-in-law is cool, calm and somewhat emotionally removed from his father-in-law's situation, but very attentive, concerned and very emotionally connected to how it is affecting his wife. He has asked several questions regarding their option to withdraw support, but his wife has just listened to the conversation.

History

NOK: daughter – well-educated professional who is used to calling the shots and being in charge in an advertising agency. Not well connected to her father during childhood. Mother and father divorced when she was 3 and he moved across the country. Her mother blocked visitation as much as possible. He had seen his daughter only a handful of times between the divorce and her 12th birthday. Three days after that birthday, her mother was hit by a car while jogging and killed instantly. At that time, she went to live with her father, found that he was not a monster, and they developed a close relationship. She originally took her job because the company's location was near her father. She is married to a corporate lawyer, but he is definitely the second man in her life.

Donor/patient – Financial manager who did well and ultimately started buying, rebuilding and selling small, then mid-sized and later large companies. He surprised everyone, including his daughter, when he decided to retire early and live off his sizable fortune and investments. He immediately took some time to sail around the world solo and then began to dabble in the world of personal fitness and wound up starting a business in that arena, then another and another. He was, again, involved with day-to-day operations and all the stress that brings. His daughter was worried about his stress level and had suggested the marathon training to get his mind off the business and his head out in the morning air. Patient has no regular girlfriend or much social life – when he is not working, he takes care of mowing and gardening at his modest home. He has two Labradors (a black and a yellow) and a fish tank.

Social history

See above.

Challenge statements/questions

Daughter: (Use whatever fits in the moment – but should be short statements bracketed by looking down and crying at times) 'It's *my* fault, I should have known better than challenge him to do this!' 'Would he had been O.K. if I hadn't made him run this morning?' 'Who *are* you anyway?' 'He looks fine, just like he's sleeping.' 'My mom is already dead, he can't die too.' 'What's your company?'

Son-in-law: 'She can't stand much more of this!' 'Can't someone bring us some *good* news?' 'We need to get home to the kids.' 'We just want this over as soon as possible.' 'Can't you see you are hurting her?' 'Can we get her a sedative?' 'Why wait until he's brain dead?' 'So you want his organs before he's dead?'

Scenario – Family Support Coordinator role

An effective approach will include questions about the family understanding the situation and have them talk about the physician's discussion with them – maybe with an offer of getting the physician again if needed. The FSC needs to make sure that the family is clear that this is unsurvivable and that brain death will most likely be the ultimate outcome. There should be some attempt to connect by seeking to know the patient and relationship – these should not be rebuffed, but answers should be limited. The FSC ultimately needs to connect well enough to ask the NOK to wait for brain death declaration and provide for medical support to keep the possibility of donation on the table.

SP's responsibilities (react and select 'What works in the moment')

Challenge the FSC by:

1. Having them explain brain death – they *should* offer to get an MD, but you should refuse and ask them to explain it. They should be clear that your loved-one is *not* brain dead at this time, although that is the expected outcome. Ask any realistic questions that you might have about the subject and watch for clarity and comfort level in the explanation.

2. Being 'all about' donation and wanting to do it 'with all your being', at which time the FSC should make sure that you understand this is a *potential* donation at this time.

3. Asking what kind continuing support really means or how long brain death takes (no-one knows as each situation is unique) or something similar.

4. Asking why the brain swells and why that is so bad. Feign as much clinical ignorance as possible but exhibit some curiosity. 'Why does ____ happen?' 'What does that mean?' The FSC should give some reasonable explanation of the physiology of brain injuries and why pressure in the skull is deadly, and be comfortable doing so – using plain language and exhibiting patience (when you are purposively trying that patience).

Information for the FSC

You were called by the ICU nurse.

Jay Collins, aged 61, was challenged by his only daughter earlier this year to train for and participate in a marathon. They were running early this morning when he grabbed his head, screamed and almost immediately lost consciousness. He has a massive bleed and will not survive. He occasionally breathes over the vent but has no other reflexes, and the neurologist expects him to progress to brain death within 24 hours – probably sooner. This has been relayed to the NOK, who is the daughter. His pressure is dropping slowly and since he is a DNR, the neurologist is reluctant to add medications to support for donation unless the family specifically authorizes it.

Mr Collins has no other family and only his daughter, Julie Smith, and her husband Dave have

been on the unit. They haven't left since their arrival 5 hours ago and have refused any attempts by social workers and chaplains to provide support. The RN says that the daughter is quite tearful and believes this situation is her fault. He also said that she seems to understand the gravity of the situation and feels that they will probably decide to withdraw support. Her husband is highly concerned over his wife and is trying to protect her in any way possible. He is functioning as interpreter and go-between for his wife and staff. He also has expressed his concerns of leaving his father-in-law on life support and dragging this out, which he does not want for his wife.

Mr Collins is not in the Donate Life Registry.

Please speak with the family regarding pressure support for Mr Collins in order to keep the option of donation open as he progresses to brain death.

Table 21.2 Example communication items from assessment checklist.

Did the FSC work to/or gain an emotional connection with NOK by their 'being' or their questions/actions? *This is your gut-level, subjective assessment*	Definitely Yes ☐	Probably Yes ☐	Not Sure ☐	Probably No ☐	Definitely No ☐
Which of the following *most* contributed to your rating? *You may check as many/none that apply*	a. Did the FSC encourage the NOK to tell his/her story? ☐ b. Did the FSC verbally or non-verbally cue the NOK to continue his/her story? ☐ c. Did the FSC actively respond to the NOK's story/cues and use supportive comments to demonstrate understanding, respect and support? ☐ d. Were the FSC's tone of voice and body language appropriate for the encounter? ☐ e. None of the above ☐				

selecting the right SPs. We found an additional consideration for selecting the right SP for this activity – the attitude of the SP towards organ donation. SPs who had strong feelings opposing organ donation – no matter how experienced or how objective they thought they could be in role – consistently impacted the role both during the activity and in feedback. It also affected the SP after the role in emotional and personal manifestations. We learned to explore those

attitudes prior to inviting the SP to be part of the activity.

Debriefing of the SP and simulated HCP after the activity became mandatory for all SPs. Providing them with a venue to switch from their in-role persona and become part of the overall activity assessment was important to diffuse any residual emotions that the SPs were feeling. This investment of time and support protected the emotional health of the SPs and ensured a greater return rate for the SPs in future activities.

This programme is a popular activity for SPs. It allows them to step outside the typical patient role and address emotional feelings about death and related issues such as do-not-resuscitate (DNR), living wills and organ donation. Many SPs self-reported a greater level of understanding of the delicate relationship between healthcare providers, the FSC and families and death. They felt that the training provided had a dramatic impact on many people – the FSC and the people who receive the organs.

Part 5
Conclusion

22 The future of simulated patient methodology

Margaret Bearman and Debra Nestel
Monash University, Clayton, Australia

OVERVIEW

This chapter summarizes our views of current and future advances in simulated patient (SP) methodology. We advocate for SP methodology being underpinned by a professional workforce, with increasingly complex, challenging and nuanced practices. We discuss some of the tensions in the SP methodology when those who are portraying roles are also examining, lecturing or supervising learners and suggest that this is an important area for future research. The chapter proposes that significant opportunities for enhanced patient-centred practice will be achieved by the inclusion of real patients in scenario development and the increasing presence of SP methodology in practice environments. Finally, we describe a range of shifting boundaries, technological and pedagogical, before suggesting 'simulated participant' (SP) as a more inclusive term.

Introduction

SPs methodology comprises a diverse collection of approaches, underpinned by theory, evidence and expert practice. As editors, we have been delighted to work with so many wonderful authors, who explore the extraordinary breadth of this interactive, immersive and effective form of simulation. This final chapter charts a future vision and draws together some of themes that run through this book.

In Chapter 8, McNaughton and Hodges described the current discourses of SP methodology in health professional education as competence, performance measurement and patient-centred care. As the diversity and depth of this book illustrate, it might be argued that an emerging discourse is that of *complexity*. SP practices are increasingly associated with a view of health professional education as intricate, interlocking systems of affordances and constraints. In this ultimate chapter, we draw upon this idea of complexity to explore some of the exciting futures of SP practice.

A spectrum of SP practices

Nestel *et al.*, Thisthlethwaite and Ridgway and Snow in Chapters 2, 3 and 14 outline the range of SP practices, from basic to advanced. There will always be a role for SPs in the development of basic skills, but we believe that more SPs will be extended to increasingly advanced practices. Many of the SP skills described in this book, such as developing scenarios, emotionally expressive portrayals, *in situ* improvisations and giving feedback, are complex and challenging practices. They require nous, thoughtfulness, a good memory and a capacity to adapt to learners' changing and unpredictable needs. Some performance studies programmes already offer modules in SP methodology and in the future this may become requisite for this type of advanced practice.

In Chapter 4, Nestel *et al.* shifted the focus from SPs to those who *educate* or *train* them – a role we will now refer to as the *SP practitioner*. Many SP practitioners already hold permanent faculty appointments, with significant teaching contributions. However, as we hope the chapters

Simulated Patient Methodology: Theory, Evidence and Practice, First Edition. Edited by Debra Nestel and Margaret Bearman.
© 2015 John Wiley & Sons, Ltd. Published 2015 by John Wiley & Sons, Ltd.

on theoretical perspectives elucidate, scholarship also underpins the professional SP canon. Likewise, the simulation research literature both draws from and influences SP methodology. We believe that the professionalization of SP practitioners is accelerating; SP practitioners are increasingly active in teaching, scholarship and research. For example, at the Standardized Patient Program, University of Toronto, there is a cohort of experienced SP educators who independently teach patient-centred communication skills at all levels of training and across many professions. They also undertake research independently and in collaboration with health professional education scholars. Likewise, the Health University of Applied Sciences in Lausanne, Switzerland, has a particular training and emerging research focus on interprofessional SP methodology. As a consequence of the research–teaching nexus, leading SP practitioners will continue to extend the boundaries of SP expertise and practice. As SP practitioners work more closely with those who teach with alternative simulation modalities (e.g. manikins), there is likely to be advancement of the methodology of all simulation practitioners.

Portraying a patient

We have situated much of our work (see Chapters 9 and 10) in the patient-centred discourse of SP methodology. For example, we repeatedly argue for a view of SPs being proxies for real patients and to provide a better understanding of the patient experience. In contrast, some SPs in high-stakes examinations in North America follow careful decision rules to make judgements on medical student performance. In this view, the SP is a patient-examiner or proxy for clinical assessors. As Chapter 7 by Murtagh describes and has been argued by others(1), the SP-as-examiner inverts the more expected dominance of the healthcare practitioner and inverts the normal form of the professional–patient power relationship. This type of status inversion also takes place when clinicians or lecturers also assume the role of patients. The tensions in these practices highlight that learning from SP methodology is contextually bound; it also reminds us that SPs are *not* real patients. Further research is needed to understand better the impact of an SPs' multiple roles – examiner, patient proxy, clinical expert

and/or communication skills expert – on learners and learning.

We believe the opportunity for real patients either to write or to collaborate in writing roles and scenarios will be a 'game changer'. As Snow describes in Chapter 14, the patients and the clinicians may not share the same understanding of good practice; and SP methodology provides the platform for exploring these differences. We argue that this conversation between the provider perspective and the patient perspective is not just for pre-qualification students, but also for practitioners. There is enormous potential for SP methodology in postgraduate environments. The focus here is on continual learning, where health professionals can develop new skills through understanding the impact that their actions has on their patients or clients in their care. In Chapter 16, Rethans and Derkx describe how incognito SPs can assist health professionals to maintain, and improve, a patient-centred approach to real clinical settings.

Shifting boundaries

The scope of SP practice is constantly expanding. The 'hybrid' simulation described by Nestel *et al.* in Chapter 2 is increasingly part of the everyday repertoire of SP practitioners. Technological development brings the promise of new opportunities for SP practice. We are likely to see innovative forms of blended simulation, with SPs working with a range of new technologies such as virtual environments or new simulators. SP practitioners are working more closely with simulationists who specialize in teaching with other simulation modalities. This is likely to advance all healthcare simulation education and result in a blurring of boundaries.

There will also be shifts in the location of SP practice. As more simulation is provided in real healthcare environments, at point of practice, more SP encounters will occur *in situ*. Simultaneously, mobile simulations, such as the movable operating theatre of distributed simulation(2), offer exciting opportunities for immersive simulation-based education whenever and wherever it is needed. Again, technology will increasingly alter the experience of learners and SPs alike. As Rethans and Derkx outline in Chapter 16, SP encounters can take place over the telephone, an old technology. Newer technologies provides opportunities to explore new ways of providing feedback via audiovisual capture and 'remote' assessment(3–5). Increased web-based delivery of SP training and of resources for students(6) and distance learners at all levels of training will become a familiar part of the SP methodology landscape. It is critical, however, that technology does not obscure the advantages that a living, responsive SP brings to role portrayal.

Shifts in educational practice will also influence SP methodology in unforeseen ways; new forms of formative and summative assessment may alter the future scope of SP practice. The developing interplay between SP methodology and both simulation-based education in specific and health professional education in general, highlights the potential value of an SP practitioner with educational, simulation and communication skills expertise. There is enormous untapped potential to improve teamwork and interprofessional practice through SP methodology. In a future that is increasingly focused on interdisciplinary care, the unique insights that an SP can bring from the patient experience but also from a general educational perspective (both 'inside' and 'outside' the team), is even more important.

These developments will not be without new challenges. Vnuk in Chapter 11 emphasized the importance of caring for SPs involved in physical examination. As SPs take on more demanding practices, vigilance will be necessary to ensure their psychological safety. Ethical issues and patient confidentiality will become more important in SP methodology as SPs work more in clinical settings and directly with real patients. New types of 'contracts' may need to be formed between faculty, practitioners, learners and SPs.

Standing at the cusp of this future, we believe that it is timely to reconsider the term 'simulated patient'. Many health professions refer to the 'client', 'service user' or 'team member' rather than 'patient'. Additionally, SP roles can include family members and healthcare professionals; the line between the 'confederate' and SP is almost entirely semantic. SPs may also work in communication skills training beyond healthcare, as a range of different sectors, including the legal and corporate sectors, also have requirements. The term, 'simulated participant' may better reflect these extended roles.

Conclusion

From thinking about the complexity of SP practice, it is worth ending with a note about its simplicity. At its core, SP methodology is about learning through the experience of interacting with others. The current value of SP methodology to healthcare practice cannot be understated. There are thousands of healthcare practitioners today who can describe a formative moment in their education, which took place as a consequence of an SP encounter. This book celebrates this achievement.

References

1 Hanna M and Fins JJ (2006) Viewpoint: power and communication: why simulation training ought to be complemented by experiential and humanist learning. *Academic Medicine*, **81**(3): 265–70.

2 Kneebone R, Arora S, King D, Bello F, Sevdalis N, Kassab E, *et al.* (2010) Distributed simulation – accessible immersive training. *Medical Teacher*, **32**(1): 65–70.

3 Kneebone R, Nestel D, Ratnasothy J, Kidd J and Darzi A (2003) The use of handheld computers in scenario-based procedural assessments. *Medical Teacher*, **25**(6): 632–42.

4 Kneebone R, Bello F, Nestel D, Mooney N, Codling A, Yadollahi F, *et al.* (2008) Learner-centred feedback using remote assessment of clinical procedures. *Medical Teacher*, **30**: 795–801.

5 Nestel D, Bello F, Kneebone R and Darzi A (2008) Remote assessment and learner-centred feedback using the Imperial College Feedback and Assessment System (ICFAS). *The Clinical Teacher*, **5**: 88–92.

6 Lax L, Russel IL, Nelles L and Smith C (2009) Scaffolding knowledge building in a web-based communication and cultural competence program for international medical graduates. *Academic Medicine*, **84**(10 Suppl.): S5–8.

Index

Printed and bound by CPI Group (UK) Ltd, Croydon, CR0 4YY
14/05/2021
03072878-0001